ELDER CARE CATASTROPHE

D1466659

ELDER CARE CATASTROPHE

RITUALS OF ABUSE IN NURSING HOMES— AND WHAT YOU CAN DO ABOUT IT

JASON S. ULSPERGER AND
J. DAVID KNOTTNERUS

Paradigm Publishers
Boulder • London

Copyright © 2011 Paradigm Publishers

Published in the United States by Paradigm Publishers, 2845 Wilderness Place, Boulder, CO 80301 USA.

Paradigm Publishers is the trade name of Birkenkamp & Company, LLC, Dean Birkenkamp, President and Publisher.

Library of Congress Cataloging-in-Publication Data

Ulsperger, Jason S.
  Elder care catastrophe : rituals of abuse in nursing homes—and what you can do about it / Jason S. Ulsperger and J. David Knottnerus.
    p. cm.
  Includes bibliographical references and index.
  ISBN 978-1-59451-906-2 (hardcover : alk. paper)
  ISBN 978-1-59451-907-9 (pbk. : alk. paper)
  1. Nursing home care. 2. Nursing home patients—Abuse of. 3. Older people—Nursing home care. 4. Older people—Abuse of. I. Knottnerus, J. David. II. Title.
RA997.U44 2010
362.16—dc22
                                                                              2010017991

Printed and bound in the United States of America on acid-free paper that meets the standards of the American National Standard for Permanence of Paper for Printed Library Materials.

Designed and Typeset by Straight Creek Bookmakers

15 14 13 12 11 1 2 3 4 5

We dedicate this book to all nursing home residents who have suffered from the unanticipated consequences of bureaucracy and all of the nursing home employees who have to juggle work tasks and emotional well-being while trapped in the iron cage.

CONTENTS

PREFACE

We met ten years ago on the campus of Oklahoma State University. One of us was teaching a graduate-level social theory course. The other was a wide-eyed student taking the course in one of his first years of graduate school after deciding not to become a nursing home administrator following some time working at a facility in northeast Arkansas. In the course, one topic covered was bureaucracy—the organizational type sociologist Max Weber argued leads to the objectification of people with its focus on staff separation, rules, documentation, and efficiency. Outside of class, we discussed the bureaucratic dynamics that apply to nursing home life and our own experiences with loved ones and long-term care. Those conversations led to a series of research projects. Nine years later, we decided to write a book called *Elder Care Catastrophe* based on our academic investigations and personal experiences with nursing homes.

Nursing homes have been around for many decades. While family and friends still provide a majority of elder care, nursing homes remain a relevant component of the long-term care industry. Although alternatives to nursing homes currently exist, including assisted living and home health services, many elderly people who cannot age in place for various reasons still end up in nursing homes. That makes problems surrounding nursing home care highly relevant, especially with the baby boom generation entering retirement age.

C. Wright Mills (1959) argued that it is essential for us to use our "sociological imaginations" to recognize that public issues help to explain much of our personal troubles. Unfortunately, we live in a time when people like to point the finger at individuals when explaining the consequences of social problems. The existence of nursing home neglect and abuse is no exception. We use the Mills perspective throughout this book to argue that bureaucratic ritualized practices facilitate much of the maltreatment occurring in nursing homes. The book starts with chapters reviewing nursing home neglect and abuse, the growth of bureaucracy, the history of nursing homes, and themes of bureaucracy relating to nursing home maltreatment. It then provides a systematic categorization of different forms of nursing home mistreatment, including chapters on emotional neglect, physical maltreatment, and verbal abuse. In a subsequent chapter, we detail what we call the CARE model—a systematic set of recommendations to lessen aspects of resident neglect and abuse in nursing homes. The book concludes with a chapter discussing how nursing home neglect and abuse is part of a larger bureaucratic catastrophe.

We believe the book can be beneficial to a variety of people, including academicians, whether they are interested in gerontology, organizational analysis, or sociology. We also think policy makers, especially those with an interest in political issues on long-term care, can increase their understanding of nursing home issues by reading this book. We hope people who work in nursing homes, from front-line staff to top administrators, will benefit from the bureaucratic awareness provided by *Elder Care Catastrophe*. Finally, we anticipate that potential residents, current residents, and family members of residents will gain considerable insights on nursing homes by reading the book and reviewing the appendices, which include recommendations on nursing home selection.

In closing, we would like to thank all those people who contributed information for this book. This includes a variety of nursing home residents and their family members, as well as people working in nursing homes. We also thank Cole Smith and Ashley Lumpkin for the information we used that came from their interviews. Kristen Ulsperger did a great deal of reading and editing for this project, and she deserves recognition for it. Finally, we would like to acknowledge the help of Bernard Phillips, who spearheaded the formation of the Sociological Imagination Group. He provided us with a great deal of extremely valuable advice and has from the very start strongly supported and encouraged our writing of this work. We would also like to thank Dean Birkenkamp, Paradigm's publisher, who has also been particularly helpful and supportive of this project. We are truly indebted to all of these people.

Jason S. Ulsperger   *J. David Knottnerus*
Department of Behavioral Sciences   *Department of Sociology*
Arkansas Tech University   *Oklahoma State University*

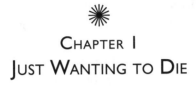

Chapter 1
Just Wanting to Die

In a hospital they throw you out into the street
before you are half cured, but in a nursing home
they don't let you out till you are dead.
                    George Bernard Shaw

A nursing home bus crushed Mary C. Knight. With her body behind the left rear tire, the driver shifted into reverse. According to the driver, something felt like it was keeping her from backing up. She was right. It was Mary's left arm and back. The Benton, AR, nursing home resident had just arrived at a vocational program affiliated with her long-term care facility, Arkansas Health Center, when the incident took place. Somehow, staff lost track of where she was after the bus unloaded. According to Arkansas' Office of Long Term Care, someone heard Mary say the day before that she wanted to die (Managed Care Weekly 2004; Smith 2005).

The courts ordered the elderly Knight to the supervision of Arkansas Health Center after finding her incapable of living in mainstream society. Psychiatrists diagnosed her with dementia, bipolar disorder, and alcohol-dependence issues. Based on these issues, it seems Mary's death might have been a suicide, a position held by the Arkansas Health Center. However, Mary's ex-husband thinks differently. He decided to sue the facility, the state of Arkansas, and the vocational program operating under the nursing home's trust. His attorney believes litigation is necessary because, "Anyone who suggests that this lady was distraught or depressed or suicidal overlooks the fact that she was also committed involuntarily to that institution." He goes on, "One of the things that you have to do when the state has custody of someone who's incompetent and insane is they've got to take care of them" (Smith 2005).

Mary's death was another in a long line of mysterious deaths at Arkansas Health Center. In a period of one year, five deaths associated with employee mistakes occurred at the institution. Other questionable events cited by nursing home investigators included staff ritualistically neglecting privacy by failing to knock on resident doors when entering and allowing resident catheter tubes to drag the floor. Again, those were the cited issues. A couple of years before her death, Mary was involved in an undocumented instance involving poor employee supervision. She left a work therapy building on the grounds and came up missing. Someone eventually found her lying on the ground with her pants pulled down. A male resident was allegedly kneeling over her with his penis exposed (Managed Care Weekly 2004).

Unfortunately, incidents such as Mary's are not rare. They are just a couple of examples of the many acts of neglect and abuse that happen in U.S. nursing homes every year. While elder abuse is common in nursing homes, we do not think it is always something employees want to happen. We believe that in a nursing home's daily grind, which includes large numbers of rules, regulations, and paperwork, goals for providing compassionate care get lost. In turn, many forms of neglect and abuse occur. Family members, researchers, and policy makers need to start seriously turning their attention to this social problem. This chapter starts building your understanding of America's elder care catastrophe by discussing elderly population growth, the long-term-care continuum, and the growth of maltreatment in nursing homes. It concludes with an outline briefly stating the purpose of each remaining chapter in the book.

The Age Wave

To understand the relevance of nursing home maltreatment, it is important to know that the United States, a once young country, is getting old. Dychtwald refers to this population shift as the "age wave" (1999:57). The average person in the United States now has more living parents than children and an American woman spends more time caring for her parents than for her own kids (Riekse and Holstege 1996), all because the population aged 65 and older is growing at its most rapid rate ever.

Although it seems strange now, in colonial times, most of the American population was under the age of 16. Many did not make it to old age. Even up until 1900, life expectancy at birth in the United States was around 50 years (Bova and Noble 2007). Two factors kept the population young: elevated fertility rates and high rates of mortality. However, both of these factors flipped during the twentieth century, and a movement occurred involving the desire to control aging processes. The result of these factors was a demographic quake: The winds of aging shifted and the age wave emerged.

Fertility-Rate Shifts

Fertility is the ability to produce children. At the dawn of the twentieth century, the fertility rate was high, with an average of seven births per woman. By the end of the century, it dropped to two births per woman (U.S. Bureau of the Census 1993). People started having fewer children for a variety of reasons. There were more opportunities for women outside of the home and having a multitude of children to care for at home limited those opportunities. Medical advances such as the birth control pill provided women with reliable options for pregnancy prevention (Quadagno 2008). However, the biggest influence on fertility and the age wave involved baby boomers. The shift from a birthing to an aging culture gained momentum after World War II. Millions of service personnel returned from overseas. These soldiers met young women in waiting and the result was an explosion in births. Between 1946 and 1964, the number of births was 70 percent greater than in the previous two decades (U.S. Bureau of the Census 1993).

The baby boom put a large strain on institutions. When boomers reached school age, there was a shortage of schools for them. Hospitals could not meet increased demands for child health care. Dwellings such as apartments did not have enough bedrooms for kids. Baby food ran low, diapers were scarce, and stores could not keep enough toys stocked. When birth rates declined, people realized that the baby boom generation would be a concern at every stage of life. When they reached early adulthood, college enrollments swelled. In the 1970s, they purchased homes and the increased demand prompted a rise in prices. The average cost of a new home went from $26,000 to about $47,000. The power of baby boomers continues to influence American life. Some people think that boomers will sway most political and consumer decisions made in this century (Dychtwald 1999; Quadagno 2008; Siegel 1993).

Mortality Transitions

Mortality involves likelihood of death. In 1900, the chance of dying young was high and the odds of living to old age were low. Around

20 percent of white children and 30 percent of nonwhite children died before turning five. About 60 percent of white females and 30 percent of nonwhite females reached the age of 60. Only half of white males and nearly 30 percent of nonwhite males could expect to live to 60. Now, infants in the United States have a better chance than ever to survive to old age. Whites continue to have an advantage in life expectancy over nonwhites. However, the gap is shrinking. Reaching the age of 60 now is possible for around 90 percent of white males and females. Slightly more than 90 percent of nonwhite females and 80 percent of nonwhite males reach 60 (Serow, Sly, and Wrigley 1990; U.S. Bureau of the Census 1993).

Big declines in death rates occurred in the 1940s and 1970s. During the 1940s, medical technology led to gains against infant and maternal mortality. In other words, more children lived past birth and more mothers made it through the birthing process. In the 1970s, death rates from heart disease declined because of prevention and treatment methods. People were smoking less than before, and new prescription drugs controlled high blood pressure. People were healthier and segments of the population expanded. This included the elderly. In fact, the fastest growing population group is now people 85 years old and older (Quadagno 2008; Treas 1995).

In 1900, 122,000 people aged 85 and older lived in the United States. At the turn of the millennium, that number increased to more than 3 million, and estimates indicate that it will reach nearly 6.5 million by 2020. The number of people over the age of 100 is also increasing at a rapid rate. In 1879, the odds of living to 100 were only 400 to 1. In 1980, the odds increased to 81 to 1. Now, there are more than 50,000 people aged 100 years and older in the United States. With advancing technology, we expect those numbers to continue to rise. The United States will soon have the largest elderly population in the world (Bova and Noble 2007; Riekse and Holstege 1996; Spencer, Goldstein, and Taeuber 1987).

Controlling Aging

We are on the verge of touching the outer limits of the human life span thanks to what we identify as the age control movement. Five breakthroughs continue to push this late-twentieth-century movement. They include super-nutrition, hormone replacement, gene therapy, bionics, and organ cloning.

Super-nutrition involves a diet rich in nutrients but low in calories. A correlation between specific food ingredients and disease prevention indicates that vitamins C and E, beta-carotene, and selenium can reinforce the immune system and prevent heart disease and even cancer (Dychtwald 1999). Hormone replacement involves supplying hormones for which a person is deficient. Regelson (1996) indicates that hormones injected into the body can slow and even stop the aging process. People use estrogen, testosterone, and human growth hormone as hormone supplements. Gene therapy focuses on changing cellular clocks found at the tips of chromosomes, which scientists call telomeres (Lewis 1998). Cells rejuvenate at astronomical rates when they are genetically changed. When dividing, the potential to increase the life span of aging cells exists. This allows an increase in human life span (Bova and Noble 2007). Bionics involves the use of artificial limbs and organs. Cloning involves the creation of human tissue in a laboratory setting and has the ability to benefit elderly people with brain diseases or cancer patients needing healthy cells (Dychtwald 1999).

With these technologies, by the end of the twentieth century life expectancy reached 76 years for males and 83 for females. The average American who lives to age 50 can expect to live even longer than that (Bova and Noble 2007). Regardless of medical breakthroughs, not all people reaching old age will be able to care for themselves. We cannot yet take a human brain and transplant it into a mechanical body in order to function beyond our physical limitations as humans. With the current pace of technology, we wonder if that possibility is far off. Regardless, many of the elderly still require intensive supervision due to cognitive impairment and severe health problems. Coupled with the age wave, we believe this will prompt a rise in the demand for elderly services all along the long-term-care continuum (Ulsperger and Ulsperger 2002).

The Long-Term-Care Continuum

Long-term care involves a range of health supervision, personal care, and social services given over a lengthy amount of time for people who cannot care for themselves. Informal long-term care, which friends and relatives give, is the most common form (Montgomery 1992). The common belief that Americans focus on youth and autonomy while disregarding the needs of the aged is a myth. In the United States, young family members still provide a majority of care for their elderly loved ones (Brody 1984, 1990).

American women provide most informal long-term care for the elderly. Indeed, more than 70 percent of long-term care providers are female family members (Stone, Cafferata, and Sangl 1987). These women pay a high emotional price because women have a hard time distancing themselves from caregiving (Zarit, Todd, and Zarit 1986). Family obligations do lead to care by younger generations, but we think the use of formal long-term care will increase because family size is shrinking and more women are spending time in the labor market (Cicirelli 1990).

Formal Long-Term Care

For people who do not have the capability to care for an aged loved one, a nursing home does not have to be the first option. A variety of alternatives exists, including home care, adult day care, respite care, and assisted living. If a nursing home does not seem right for your situation, any of these programs might fit your level of need.

Home care refers to in-home health and supportive services. This includes professional, paraprofessional, and long-term care in a recipient's home. Home care is hard to define because it includes a wide range of services. For example, it includes physician and nurse visits as well as house-cleaning services. The use of home-based services is not widespread. At the end of the twentieth century, only three percent of the elderly in the United States reported using a visiting nurse and two percent used home health services and home-delivered meals (Montgomery 1992; Stone 1986). However, the use of such services is increasing (Marrelli and Whittier 2008).

Adult day care involves community programs that provide services to older people. They usually run in daytime hours. Adult day-care facilities vary in terms of emphasis, but two primary models exist. The first is the health rehabilitative model, which offers medical, nursing, and therapy services. The second type is the social psychological model, which involves people recovering from illness and those who typically have dementia. Adult day cares are located in a variety of settings. Charging by the hour and by the day, they operate in churches, senior centers, and hospitals (Giacalone 2001; Montgomery 1992). More than 1,000 exist in the United States averaging a daily enrollment of 24 people (Conrad, Hanrahan, and Hughes 1990; Richardson, Dabelko, and Gregoire 2008).

Respite care involves planned relief. It allows people to drop off elder family members at a facility. With these services, you can essentially pay for hourly temporary care to get a break from the exhaustion that can occur when taking care of a loved one. Family caregivers often show declines in physical and mental health due to chronic fatigue, isolation, and financial stress. Through respite care services, caregivers can take time out to pursue personal interests and relaxation (Mace and Rabins 2006; Scharlach and Frenzel 1986).

Assisted-living facilities are for non-impaired elders needing help with some activities of daily living such as food preparation, bathing, and medications. People in these facilities do not need 24-hour care. They receive meals in a common dining room, but have separate lodging and housekeeping services. Assisted-living facilities have a small staff of at least one nurse, a social worker, and a case manager. They contract health care services to external agencies, which keeps costs low. Often, people in these facilities pay with private funds (Giacalone 2001; Seipke 2008). If you or your aged loved one is not financially secure enough to afford assisted living, or if your elderly loved one needs a higher level of supervision, you might have to consider nursing home options.

The Nursing Home as Long-Term Care

Nursing homes provide a majority of formal long-term care. They treat patients with chronic illnesses. Although they provide less intensive care than general hospitals, they do have trained nursing staff. Medicare and Medicaid certify nursing homes as eligible for reimbursement based on the type of care provided. More than 95 percent of nursing homes receive government reimbursements. By doing so, they subject themselves to inspections carried out by state officials. In addition to providing elders who cannot care for themselves a place to live, nursing homes provide help with what people in the industry call activities of daily living, or ADLs. This includes assistance with anything from dressing to bathing. Nearly 50 percent of people who live in nursing homes have dementia. In fact, more facilities than ever now exclusively serve cognitively impaired populations or have at least one designated area that focuses on them. For example, many nursing homes have Alzheimer's wings (Carlson and Hsiao 2006; Kahana and Brittis 1992). The average cost for a private room in a nursing home is currently $75,190 per year. A shared room with a partition between the beds averages $66,795 per year (MetLife 2006).

Through the 1980s, levels of care at nursing homes ranged from certified skilled nursing facilities (SNFs) to intermediate care facilities (ICFs). SNFs provided supervision 24 hours per day for residents under the care of a registered nurse. Like assisted living facilities, ICFs provided lower levels of care (Sirrocco 1989). After the Omnibus Budget Reconciliation Act of 1987, also known as the Nursing Home Reform Act, the distinction between SNFs and ICFs blurred. Most agencies now classify all of these institutions as nursing facilities (Carlson and Hsiao 2006; Richardson 1990). Regardless, do not get perplexed over names. As some analysts point out, when facilities do not want people to recognize them as "nursing homes," they will actively promote other names to avoid any stigma associated with the nursing home label. This can be anything from health care facility to rehabilitation center (for more on this phenomenon see Ulsperger and Paul 2002). To avoid confusion, throughout this book, we simply use the term nursing home.

Facility and Resident Numbers

The number of nursing homes in the United States peaked in 1985, with slightly more than 19,000 facilities. Then new ways of care previously mentioned, such as home health care and assisted living, started replacing services provided by nursing homes and the number of facilities declined. In addition, disability rates for the elderly lowered the number of aged people entering nursing homes. This trend did not last long. Reports indicate that the number of nursing homes was on the rise again in the 1990s. In 1991, the number of nursing homes in the United States neared 16,000 facilities. The Centers for Disease Control, which monitors nursing home health statistics, indicates the number is currently 16,100. Moreover, the presence of the "old-old," people 85 and older, in society is starting to increase disability prevalence among the elderly again, possibly setting the stage for another sharp increase in the number of nursing homes in the United States (Lakdawalla and Philipson 2002; Gabrel 2000; National Center for Health Statistics 2006; Strahan 1997).

Regardless of national trends, nursing homes themselves are getting larger. Consider the average number of beds per facility. It increased from 75 in the early 1970s, to 107 in 1997. As of 2004, 40 percent of nursing homes had 100 beds or more. Although there may be fewer nursing homes than at the industry's peak, the ones that exist are bigger than ever. The actual number of residents per facility also increased over the past few decades, receding a little only recently. In the early 1970s, a little more than one million people lived in nursing homes. By 1997, the number was 1,608,700, dipping slightly to 1,492,200 by 2004 (National Center for Health Statistics 1988, 2000, 2006).

Many people assume that most of the elderly live in nursing homes. We want to emphasize that this is a fallacy. The true number of the elderly living in nursing homes is around 4 percent. However, this figure is a little misleading. Nearly 25 percent of people over the age of 65 will spend time in a nursing home, so the likelihood of an older person's admission is high. The number, 4 percent, is also cross-sectional. It does not take into account movement in and out of nursing homes (Hooyman and Kiyak 1996; Pandya 2001). We can point out that the most common reasons for nursing home admission are circulatory disease and cognitive impairment. Problems related to cardiovascular issues, such as a stroke and its related effects, comprise 17 percent of new admissions relating to circulatory disease. The main cognitive problem relating to admission is symptoms of Alzheimer's disease (Sahyoun et al. 2001). Keep in mind, if you ever have an elderly loved one in a nursing home, the facility may not exclusively cater to the aged. Younger people with serious health problems relating to ADLs may live in the facility as well. Nonetheless, the average age of admission for elderly residents into a nursing home is 83, up from 81 just a few years ago. Approximately 88 percent of nursing home residents are elderly, with 50 percent over the age of 85. Close to 90 percent of residents are white and just over 70 percent are females (Giacalone 2001; Houser 2007; National Center for Health Statistics 2000; Sahyoun et al. 2001).

Ownership Trends

In relation to ownership, in 1986, only ten publicly held nursing home chains existed. These for-profit businesses owned and leased 170,000 beds. Though the number of nursing homes dipped for a period, the number of nursing home chains has grown. The current top ten chains account for nearly 300,000 of the nursing home beds in the United States (Giacalone 2001). In the early 1990s, the largest chain owned slightly more than 1,000 facilities with more than 100,000 beds in its possession (Forrest, Forrest, and Forrest 1993). As of 2000, it had 67,000 employees and sales reports of $116.8 million in revenue. That chain, Beverly Enterprises Incorporated, was sold to Fillmore Capital Partners for $1.8 billion in 2005 (Burling 2007; Dun and Bradstreet 2000). Since that time, buyouts and mergers have been the rage in the industry. In May 2007, Genesis, a Pennsylvania-based long-term-care corporation, accepted a merger proposal from Formation Capital and JER Partners for $1.4 billion, beating the best offer by Fillmore. In December 2007, Carlyle Group closed a $6.3 billion buyout of nursing home operator Manor Care. For-profit nursing homes, which include facilities operated by the big chains just mentioned, comprise around 60 percent of the market, with nonprofit facilities, including government homes, accounting for the rest (Meyer 2008; National Center for Health Statistics 2006).

Some sociologists believe the increased use of for-profit care, such as that in the nursing home industry, is creating a crisis with the logic that paid care leads to poor care (see for example Glenn 2000). The basic argument is that cutting corners to increase profits is costing residents quality health care and safety. However, as we argue in this book, it is possible that the focus on bureaucracy in nursing homes, regardless of ownership status, carries just as much responsibility for promoting maltreatment.

Maltreatment in Nursing Homes

Maltreatment in nursing homes involves any deviation from predicted standards for high quality care, such as physical violence, verbal aggression, and various forms of neglect (for further elaboration see Pillemer and Moore 1990). Concern over nursing home maltreatment existed for years only to become a national issue in the 1960s (Horton et al. 1997). It was then that tales of nursing home abuse started appearing in newspapers and books (see Townsend 1971; Mendelson 1974; Vladeck 1980). Government officials sensed the rise in negative sentiments and started a series of investigations (Buhler-Wilkerson 2003).

In 1986, Congress requested that the Institute of Medicine draft a report on the quality of care in nursing homes. The report confirmed academic warnings and print media stories of problems. A follow-up study conducted by the U.S. General Accounting Office found that more than one-third of nursing homes had bad care. In reaction, Congress signed the aforementioned Omnibus

Budget Reconciliation Act of 1987, also known as the Nursing Home Reform Act. New guidelines enforced by the Health Care Financing Administration (HCFA), currently the Centers for Medicare and Medicaid Services (CMS), required homes to follow strict rules through annual inspections. The guidelines also established reforms for the treatment of residents. Since establishment of the guidelines, deficiencies recorded by the HCFA declined (Harrington and Carrillo 1999; Mooney and Greenway 1996). However, media sources continue to report maltreatment.

Convoluted Concerns or Credible Catastrophe

Headlines appearing since the turn of the century highlight the continued trend of maltreatment. They indicate "Serious Deficiencies in Nursing Homes Are Often Missed" (Pear 2008) and "Unreported Abuse Found at Nursing Homes" (Pear 2002). Others indicate "Nursing Homes in Filthy State" (Williams 2005), "Nursing Home Deaths Soar" (Amon and Zambito 2001), and "Elder Care Conditions Shocking" (McCullen 2000). Different ones report "Trial Opens in 35 Nursing Home Deaths" (Jervis 2007), "Nursing Home Neglect Adds to Health Care Nightmare" (Indo 2007), and "Nursing Home Deaths Highlight Staffing Problems" (Neal and Neal 2000). People are now concerned that the abuse of elders in nursing homes constitutes a social threat. Headlines call attention to maltreatment such as "Nursing Home Nurse Accused of Raping Comatose Patient" (Adams 2000), "Worker Charged with Assaulting Alzheimer's Patient" (Rowden 1999), and "Aide Charged in Death at Nursing Home" (Warner 1999).

Sociologist Barry Glassner (1999), in his book *The Culture of Fear*, argues that nursing home headlines such as these should be of little concern when considering bigger social issues, such as poverty and social inequality. He also states, "Even in coverage of the sorry state of many of the nation's nursing homes the root of the problems of lack of funding and inadequate oversight disappear amid overdrawn images of evil caretakers" (1999: 48). We tend to agree. Research does show that nursing home stories in newspapers often downplay systemic causes and focus on a few bad apples as the reason for many nursing home ills (see Ulsperger and Ulsperger 2002). Yet, individuals are the ones who carry out acts of maltreatment reported in newspaper stories, sensationalized or not. Considering social issues that exist outside of the realm of everyday nursing home life is important. However, as you will discover reading this book, we believe the everyday, taken-for-granted rituals that occur inside nursing homes and that influence maltreatment are just as relevant.

It would be easy to dismiss nursing home maltreatment as an exaggerated turn of the millennium moral panic, but statistics give us a reasonable belief that we are in the midst of an elder care catastrophe. For example, reports indicate around 2,500 cases of physical abuse at the hands of staff occur in U.S. nursing homes every year. Approximately 36 percent of nurses and aides indicate they witness or participate in acts of physical abuse. With psychological abuse, 40 percent of nurses and aides admit to the maltreatment of residents, and 81 percent say they have witnessed it. In the states of Georgia, Illinois, and Pennsylvania, officials investigate over 150 physical and sexual abuse allegations in nursing homes per year. More than 300,000 nursing home residents live in facilities where they are at great risk of harm. More than 460,000 complaints of elder maltreatment occur yearly, many of which involve nursing homes. And around 14,000 nursing home residents die in nursing homes due to poor treatment every three years (Billups 2006; Parker, Waichman, and Alonso 2007; General Accounting Office 2002; Help Center 2008; Nerenberg 2002; Pillemer and Moore 1990).

Most reports on nursing home maltreatment deal with recorded counts of abuse. They fail to deal with neglect as maltreatment. This book focuses on both. In addition, most nursing home maltreatment research is based on estimates. There is a legitimate reason both of these things occur. First, as we point out throughout this book, in nursing home culture the belief is that if something is not documented it did not happen. Therefore, formal claims of abuse might warrant specific written reports. However, acts of negligence, such as not dressing a resident, putting clothes on backwards, invading privacy, or ignoring pleas for help, fly under the maltreatment radar. Second, in terms of estimates, we believe nursing home maltreatment, though it is not often discussed in this way, falls under what criminologists call the "dark figure of crime" (see Biderman and Reiss 1967). This term implies that many victims fail to report crime. For example, many victims do not report rape because they fear others will blame them for getting into a bad situation. Rape victims also worry about the embarrassing processes performed to verify the crime and fear the stigma associated with being a rape victim (Williams 1984). It is easy to consider nursing home maltreatment statistics as insignificant when they reveal lower than expected counts of neglect and abuse. The "dark figure" phenomenon makes you consider things in a different light. For example, estimates indicate that nearly one million seniors are victimized in nursing homes and assisted living facilities every year (Help Center 2008). Moreover, we must remember that many residents have cognitive problems and do not even realize when victimization happens to them.

This reminds us of an unfortunate story a colleague told us recently. His son got a job in a nursing home to make ends meet. While working at the facility he witnessed other aides go into residents' rooms when other staff members were not around and close the door behind them. He reported that some of the aides were frequenting the rooms of residents with cognitive impairments. After asking around, he discovered that male aides were sexually assaulting incoherent residents knowing that they would either not have the ability to report their victimization or if they did report it other staff would view their accusations as "crazy." Some aides were even having sex with each other in the rooms of mentally incompetent residents. This kind of thing does not appear in resident charts.

Ethnographic Nursing Home Research

As news of maltreatment in nursing homes emerged throughout the 1960s, a portion of researchers in sociology and anthropology started seriously studying nursing home issues. They often used ethnographic observation techniques to examine daily nursing home culture. Much of it does not focus on neglect and abuse. However, it does reveal interesting themes in relation to maltreatment. As a reader, you need some background on it because we mention it occasionally throughout this book. We encourage you to obtain each person's original work and read it.

Erving Goffman (1961) was one the first sociologists to discuss nursing homes. Though his mention of nursing homes is brief, his idea of a nursing home as a total institution had an impact. His work describes a total institution as a place where people are isolated from the rest of society for a set period. During this isolation, they come under the control of the officials running the institution. His studies indicate that routines of the institutional structure reshape the individual. When entering a total institution, a solid break with past roles and selves occurs and the individual establishes new identities. This work indicates that issues relating to maltreatment could be the result of organizational control.

Goffman's work mentions nursing homes, but Jules Henry's (1963) research specifically focuses on them, providing a comparative view of life in nursing homes. He studied a government home along with two for-profit facilities. The government nursing home was a community institute where, according to Henry's writing, staff members were efficient and the facility was sanitary. Nonetheless, the relationship between staff and residents was poor. The for-profit nursing homes had the worst characteristics. Henry refers to one for-profit facility as the "vestibule of hell" (1963: 407). He explains that staff in the facility treated residents as a mixture between dogs, children, and lunatics.

Jaber Gubrium (1975) produced the next significant study. His research concentrates on a nursing home in the Midwest. The facility was a nonprofit, church-related institution. His work provides information pertaining to organizational dynamics based on lower level and top staff. In addition, it was one of the first works to explicitly indicate that the bureaucratic routines of caring, even in a nonprofit institution, can impede quality care. Subsequent studies of importance include Carobeth Laird's (1979) exploration of Golden Mesa. She entered this nursing home at the age of 70. As she adjusted, she recorded her experiences. Her work details the depersonalization that occurs when interacting with staff.

Jeanie Kayser-Jones's (1981) work uses observation techniques to compare a for-profit nursing home in California to a nonprofit institution in Scotland. It archives how the nonprofit home had more regard for residents' personal rights, such as privacy. In the for-profit home she observed dehumanizing situations. She witnessed staff exposing patients' genitals, bathing men and women simultaneously in the same shower room, and creating a situation in which the elderly, due to a lack of help and attention, defecated and urinated on the floor.

As a nurse and anthropologist, Bethel Powers's (1988a, 1988b) research uses a network analysis to record the strategies the elderly use in nonprofit nursing homes to construct support systems. Mary O'Brien (1989) studied a nonprofit church facility in the eastern United States. Her work indicates that the institutional orientation toward morality and faith influences residents' worldviews. It shows that a religious ideology in nursing homes influences the thought patterns of caregivers and leads to better care.

Timothy Diamond (1992) worked in a nursing home as a nursing assistant. He entered the field without revealing his motives as a researcher. He explains that the administrator would not have hired him otherwise. He asserts that the study "was forced increasingly to become a piece of undercover research" (1992: 8). His work argues that for-profit nursing homes operate under a capitalist mind set. Owners of these facilities care little about how residents are treated. He points out that from the for-profit perspective, oftentimes staff members view residents as "raw materials" (1992: 211). His findings show that nursing homes operate on a logic of commodity production only concerned with "making gray gold" (1992: 5). However, he mentions that balance sheets and bottom lines also hinder care in many nonprofit institutions.

Unlike Diamond, Nancy Foner (1994) did reveal her status as a researcher in the examination of a nonprofit state nursing home in New York. Similar to ideas used in this research, her work uses theories tied to bureaucracy to argue that demands for efficiency in state facilities impede quality of care. Specifically, organizational demands to meet regulations create caregiving dilemmas for staff. Often they desire to provide family-oriented, compassionate care. However, work rules related to time constraints and laws enforced by the state force them to focus on merely getting tasks done.

Debora Paterniti's (2000) work concerns identity construction in a for-profit nursing home. Her analysis implies that resident narratives have the ability to alter staff perceptions and treatment. She points out that habitual actions by the staff develop into embedded routines. These routines contribute to a common stock of knowledge concerning interaction with residents. Specifically, they dehumanize residents by turning them into objects of work. This research reveals that residents fight this process by building personal relationships with staff. They tell staff personal thoughts and urge them to listen to personal stories so staff will see them as human beings and not just a part of the labor process.

Thomas Edward Gass (2004) worked as an aide and director of social services for more than three years. His research details typical problems experienced by nursing home employees. For example, he points out that when he worked as an aide, he had twenty-six residents on his hall. Based on his calculations he could devote only around 17 minutes to each of them per day due to his other responsibilities.

Marian Deutschman (2005) observed both nonprofit and for-profit facilities in order to analyze nursing home culture. Her work indicates that it is possible for nursing homes to alter old attitudes that facilitate poor resident care. The key is that nursing home owners and administrators have to be vested in change and able to persuasively influence everyone from staff to residents to buy into it.

Robert Kane and Joan West (2005) use autobiographical accounts of their experiences taking care of their mother, who was at a nursing home for the last few years of her life. Their story is unique because both are educators who look at nursing home culture from both academic and professional perspectives.

Gilah Silber (2007) uses experiences as a nursing home doctor to discuss the dynamics of living and dying in nursing homes. We believe these studies provide thick descriptions that reveal multiple levels of social reality existing in U.S. nursing homes. Other ethnographic research adds to their findings (see Bennett 1980; Fontana 1977; Gubrium 1993; Hale 2005; Howsden 1981; Lopez 2006a; Poxon 2004; Richard 1986; Sass 2000; Savishinsky 1991; Shapiro 2006; Stafford 2003; Stannard 1973).

Research on Ownership Variation

We have alluded to the fact that for-profit nursing homes may have a different organizational culture than others. As indicated, with the dominance of for-profit nursing homes and frequent cases of maltreatment, researchers using methods not based in ethnography have also questioned the quality of paid care. As with a lot of quantitative research, for every study you find that says one thing, you can find one that says the opposite. A plethora of statistical studies on nursing home ownership and quality of care exist. Here, we just highlight a few.

Some statistical nursing home research indicates for-profit nursing homes have levels of care that are equal to nonprofit facilities (Brooks and Hoffman 1978; Gottesman 1974; Holmberg and Anderson 1968; Levey et al. 1973; Weisbrod and Schlesinger 1983; Winn 1974). Other research shows nonprofit institutions give better care. For example, Michael Koetting's (1980) work finds that nonprofit nursing homes provide premium care because they are more expensive and they spend more money on caring for residents. It finds for-profit homes are more efficient but less expensive. To compare the quality of care, Roberta Riportella-Muller and Doris Slesinger's (1982) research uses a bank of complaints filed with the Wisconsin Ombudsman Program, a service set up to monitor nursing home maltreatment. Specifically, it matches complaint data with government information on nursing home violations. Although the size of the nursing home has an influence, the findings suggest that nonprofit homes receive a lower number of complaints.

Frank Elwell's (1984) research examines nursing homes in New York. In the study, nonprofit homes account for 195 of the institutions examined while for-profit homes account for 298. The findings indicate that government nursing homes spend more money on daily operations. Other nonprofit homes, like those run by religious affiliations, spend a considerable amount on residents, but do not overspend. For-profit homes spend less. Research by Sonne Lemke and Rudolf Moos (1986) examines differences in nursing homes and other types of long-term care. Their findings show nursing homes are less likely to promote independent living. They also show nonprofit facilities exceed for-profit facilities on comfort and quality staff relationships. Lemke and Moos's (1989) later work finds that nonprofit and for-profit facilities have different social climates. They explain that nonprofit facilities are more likely to promote autonomy. They also give residents a greater voice in institutional policy. Moreover, nonprofit facilities provide a sense of community.

Anne Jenkins and John Braithwaite's (1993) work shows that deviations from government regulations are more likely in for-profit nursing homes. It examines Australian nursing homes. It shows neglect, the denial of human rights, and maltreatment in most nursing homes. However, for-profit homes have a higher rate of deviance based on a market mindset. The findings indicate that noncompliance emerges from senior management pressure to reach financial goals. They show that without profit as a major motive, nonprofit nursing homes have less pressure to violate regulations. This leads to better care.

Ulsperger and Ulsperger's (2001) research on nursing homes in the southern United States also indicates variety in care. It explores a sample of nursing homes from Arkansas, Oklahoma, Louisiana, and Mississippi using HCFA data. In the study, for-profit homes had more government citations. When examining each state, the analysis revealed differences in overall citations in the states of Arkansas, Oklahoma, and Louisiana. Citations for for-profit and nonprofit homes were not statistically significant in the state of Mississippi; however, the average number of citations was higher. Kelsey Simons's (2006) analysis shows that in nonprofit facilities in rural areas social service directors are more qualified compared to directors of most for-profit homes in suburban and urban areas.

Anna Amirkhanyan, Hyun Joon Kim, and Kristina Lambright's (2008) research argues that service quality and access are fundamentally different in view of nursing home ownership. It indicates that when considering all of the research, for-profit nursing homes still just do not perform well when it comes to quality resident care. Smaller, nonprofit facilities with high staff ratios, highly certified employees, and active resident councils do. In addition, facilities with specialized units for residents with dementia have lower levels of resident satisfaction (for other studies see Anderson et al. 2005; Eaton 2005; Elwell 1984; Fottler, Smith, and James 1981; Green and Monahan 1981; Hawes and Phillips 1986; Kane et al. 2004; Lucas et al. 2007).

The Purpose of This Book

To understand situations like Mary C. Knight's, this book uses a theory based on the study of everyday rituals. It provides an in-depth analysis of America's elder care catastrophe with a focus on for-profit and nonprofit nursing home neglect and abuse. Though some studies indicate the superiority of nonprofit nursing homes, we believe all nursing homes have problems. For example, strangers care for residents in both for-profit and nonprofit institutions. This creates a situation where staff, who have little emotional connection to residents, may provide poor care. Complex government regulations bombard for-profit and nonprofit nursing homes as well. This requires caregivers to spend more time on paperwork and less time with residents. In other words, bureaucratic constraints impede social and emotional activities in all facilities.

We should note that this book is part of an attempt by a group of sociologists, known as the Sociological Imagination Group, trying to revive the idea that sociology should analyze human behavior to develop solutions for social problems. As such, considering both employee and resident interaction, it focuses on more than the analysis of bureaucratic constraints. It also specifically concentrates on ritualized aspects of emotional, physical, and verbal neglect and abuse.

Outline of the Chapters

The outline of the chapters is as follows:

Chapter 2, "Bureaucracy and Rituals in Everyday Life": In this book, we explain that bureaucracy dominates nursing home interactions. This chapter discusses basic ideas associated with the concept of bureaucracy. This involves a brief review of sociological thinker Max Weber's (1946) ideas on how organizations function, in addition to producing dysfunction. Bureaucracy, from his perspective, reflects a desire to coordinate individual action with rules that promote organizational efficiency. Along with a review of bureaucracy, this chapter discusses the idea of rituals and briefly reviews the logic behind an innovative, new perspective in the social sciences known as structural ritualization theory.

Chapter 3, "A History of Nursing Homes": In order to understand a problem like nursing home maltreatment, the circumstances leading to the development of the problem must be considered. To understand how bureaucracy facilitates physical neglect in both for-profit and nonprofit nursing homes, this chapter reflects on various social and historical factors tied to the development of the nursing home industry.

Chapter 4, "Rules over Compassion": This chapter explains how demands for nursing home reform led to an array of regulations for facilities receiving government funding. These rules and regulations generated nursing homes driven by bureaucracy. This culture of bureaucracy has shaped rituals of behavior for employees and ultimately influenced the way they do their jobs. This chapter explains how daily work rituals involving rules, staff separation, documentation, efficiency, and meetings take away from the goals of care, unintentionally prompting a lower level of care for residents.

Chapter 5, "Products Not People": This chapter blends a discussion of bureaucracy and emotional neglect and abuse of nursing home residents. On the premise that employees ritualistically view residents as unemotional work products and not people, it explains the dynamics of four basic types of emotional neglect and abuse. This includes aspects of objectification, inadequate compassion, spiritual neglect, and ridicule.

Chapter 6, "Tranquilizing the Troublemakers": This chapter addresses bureaucracy and the physical neglect and abuse of nursing home residents. It details aspects of medical, personal, and environmental negligence. In addition, it discusses factors involving bodily harm, limited supplies, and inappropriate architecture.

Chapter 7, "I'm No Baby": This chapter covers bureaucracy and ritualized verbal maltreatment of nursing home residents. It concerns three types of verbal abuse. Specifically, it discusses infantilization, spoken aggression, and the ignoring of residents.

Chapter 8, "Alternatives to Bureaucracy in Nursing Homes": This chapter summarizes important points of the book. It also reviews the culture-change movement currently occurring in the nursing home industry. Building on that movement, it then discusses different techniques we believe that practitioners could implement in order to prevent nursing home abuse.

Chapter 9, "The Bureaucratic Boom: Are There Other Options?": This chapter argues that bureaucracy and its negative aspects are at the root of many social problems. Consider the bureaucratic failure associated with the September 11, 2001 terrorist attacks or the dysfunction of bureaucracy during and after the Hurricane Katrina disaster. This chapter goes beyond a discussion of bureaucracy in nursing homes and provides alternatives with the potential to alter any organization suffering from the unanticipated consequences of bureaucracy.

A note about our analysis and presentation of data: We designed this book in line with a perspective called the Web/Part Whole approach. It was developed by Bernard Phillips and others, such as Tom Scheff, who are associated with the Sociological Imagination Group (see Knottnerus and Phillips 2009; Phillips 2001, 2007, 2009; Phillips and Christner 2009; Phillips and Johnston 2007; Phillips, Kincaid, and Scheff 2002). This involves defining and linking a specific problem to other fundamental problems, moving up language's ladder of abstraction by using high-level ideas for understanding, moving down language's ladder of abstraction in obtaining facts, and integrating knowledge from specialized fields. In using this approach, we utilize previous ethnographic research, interviews, and both authors' own experiences of nursing home culture to draw attention to ritualized aspects of neglect and abuse. Chapters on bureaucratic, emotional, physical, and verbal issues include content analysis data comparing the presence of specific rituals in previous literature written about for-profit and nonprofit nursing home culture. They also include sections reflecting direct oral accounts we collected from residents, family members, and employees of nursing homes. The content analysis information dissects maltreatment issues, while the personal narratives provide firsthand, thick descriptions of nursing home culture by people who live it every day (for more on our methods see Appendix 1).

Chapter 2
Bureaucracy and Rituals
in Everyday Life

The growth of bureaucracy, both public and
private, is widely recognized as one of the major
social trends of our time.

Robert Merton

Oscar is somewhat of an angel of death. People who know him
tell you that you would never expect it. He has a youthful, clown-
ish, and sometimes disconnected personality. Regardless, he walks
the halls of Steere House Nursing and Rehabilitation Center in
Providence, RI, waiting for other residents to die. He has lived
on the third floor of the center for about three years. He will
show up at the door of a fellow resident about an hour before
that person's death. Eventually, he will position himself on the
bed, seemingly reading the body aura of the dying person. It is
then that nursing staff know it is time to call in family and pre-
pare them for the parting of their loved one. Oscar has predicted
more than 25 deaths. According to registered nurse Brenda Toll,
his methods are "kind of weird, but kind of lovely," and he has

become an accepted part of the "death ritual" at the nursing home (Nickerson 2007).

Oscar spent the early part of his life homeless. Given his special abilities, some people argue that he should have spent his early years as a funeral director with such a wonderful, yet unexplainable, gift. He is so highly regarded that Rhode Island's largest hospice gave the grayish-white-haired phenomenon an honorary certificate of accomplishment. However, not everyone is impressed with Oscar. One family refused to have him in the room when their loved one passed. Someone shut the door in his face and he angrily sat outside of the door (Brown 2007; Gifford-Jones 2007). Perhaps the most interesting thing about Oscar is that he is a cat, and he gained national prominence when the prestigious *New England Journal of Medicine* published an article about him (Dosa 2007).

What we find so interesting about Oscar's story is that he lives in a facility where trained medical staff should be more astute than a cat at recognizing the unseen humanness of death. But is this possible? We think it has less to do with the miraculous abilities of a feline and more to do with the automated, bureaucratic social worlds, such as nursing homes, that we interact in on a daily basis. In this chapter we turn our attention to the concept of bureaucracy. We also briefly review the idea of rituals and how they affect our everyday, taken-for-granted lives.

Understanding Bureaucracy

Bureaucratic organizations play a large role in society. Among a variety of things, they feed, educate, and employ us. With nursing homes, they rehabilitate and provide medical care for Americans who cannot care for themselves. With bureaucratic organizations dominating so much of our lives, what do we really know about them?

Early Conceptions

Bureaucracy is a combination of the French phrase *bureau* and the Greek term *kratia*. The former means office, the latter means rule. History tells us that bureaucratic organizational characteristics existed as far back as imperial Rome and ancient China, but a French official was the first to use the term in the seventeenth century to describe the operation of his government. Regardless, the first scholar to systematically analyze the idea was sociologist Max Weber (Hancock 2006).

In the early 1900s, Weber argued that bureaucracy was on the rise due to the progressive use of rationality and legal authority. Aspects of scientific logic were rapidly replacing supernatural perceptions of the world, along with a rise in the perceived superiority of law in the management of human interaction. Weber believed this laid the foundation for people to see the use of bureaucracy as a superior and fair way to process growing populations (Weber 1946). For example, it would be irrational, if not impossible, to have traditional, small schoolhouses meet the educational needs of contemporary U.S. children who have such diverse personal characteristics and backgrounds.

Weber believed the ideal bureaucracy has a hierarchy of offices held together with specific rules. Within each level, workers have a designated mark of competence determined by educational credentials. If they do not have the appropriate skills, they receive training. The specialized focus at each level provides for a smooth flow of work. Workers should also document nearly everything. This helps to standardize employee behavior and increase efficiency (Ryan 2005).

Weber pointed out many advantages of bureaucracies. They promote efficient people processing, as well as organizational stability, predictable and fair outcomes, and employee control. They also encourage low rates of employee discrimination since they focus on credentials and not personal characteristics and connections. Weber was also concerned to point out disadvantages. Too much structure and regulation leads to inefficiency. Here, we have the classic "cutting through red tape" complaint. Specific rules and procedures become the focus, and the organization loses sight of what it is supposed to do in the first place. We will come back to this point shortly. Weber also pointed out that the large-scale processing of people decreases the human nature of interaction. Have you ever been at the Department of Motor Vehicles, a doctor's office, or in an educational system where your identification involves numbers and not your name? Employees in those contexts often do not care much about personal problems you had that morning. They just want to know your social security number, health insurance card number, or student I.D. so they can process you as fast as possible. To them, you are not a person; you are a work product. Weber believed that employees in bureaucracies can experience alienation as a result of the dehumanized roles they play. He specifically noted that they can end up feeling like meaningless cogs in a larger machine. Weber also pointed out that bureaucracies have the potential to institutionalize discrimination into their rules and procedures, subsequently amplifying aspects of it. Finally, Weber warned that bureaucracies, for better or worse, once set into motion are nearly impossible to stop (Ryan 2005).

We think it is important to note that Weber discussed for-profit and nonprofit bureaucracy. Some people think bureaucracy only exists in government organizations. This may be due to the idea that higher accountability in the public sector creates more formal rule-based controls than the for-profit sector needs. However, research shows private-sector administrators have a higher commitment to rules and regulations and some private-sector organizations have characteristics that more closely mimic Weber's bureaucratic ideal type. While private ownership is dedicated to the accumulation of revenue, experts at each hierarchical level still have to control day-to-day operations (Allison 2007; Clegg 2007). We believe this supports our argument that bureaucracy in for-profit *and* nonprofit nursing homes is to blame in a large part for resident maltreatment.

Building on Weber

Scholars have built on Weber's ideas over the years. Robert Merton's (1936, 1940) work implies top-down pressures for reliability and predictability in organizations lead to standardized behavior. However, habitual actions lead to unanticipated consequences. As mentioned earlier, the organization loses sight of what it is supposed to do in the first place. Rules become ritualistic ends in themselves. As we discuss in this book, with bureaucratic logic in nursing homes being so prevalent, employees sometimes forget that they are there to provide quality care to residents, and instead focus too much on following institutional regulations. Merton's writings point out that a stimulus-response dynamic exists under this premise. Workers in bureaucratic environments see that leaders reward people for following rules instead of focusing on the original intent of the organization. This creates dysfunctional personalities that fixate on rule following just for raises or to move up the organizational hierarchy (Allison 2007).

Alvin Gouldner's (1954) work focuses on a gypsum manufacturing plant. It implies that bureaucratic behavior hinges just as much on informal rules. Employees develop their own guidelines. Gouldner determined that in some bureaucracies, norms on tardiness, illegally using company materials, and taking extended lunches exist. Most of us who have worked in a bureaucracy can relate to these. Regardless, he found that these indulgency patterns create problems when a bureaucracy hires new administrators. If new leaders do not accept them, high levels of conflict emerge that inhibit efficiency.

Stanley Udy's (1959) research was some of the first to be concerned with measuring specific bureaucratic characteristics. His work, which helped spawn other important studies, points out that an organization is not a bureaucracy unless it has at least three levels of authority, with members on one level subordinate to at least one person on the level above. Tom Burns and George Stalker's (1961) research focuses on the Scottish electronics industry. It finds a distinction between mechanistic and organic organizations. Mechanistic organizations are closed off from the external environment. They are stable. They also have characteristics that align with the ideal bureaucracy discussed by Weber. Organic organizations are less formal. They are open to input from the outside. They have traits that do not fit the bureaucratic mold and are, in fact, more effective when they exist in rapidly changing markets.

Richard Hall's (1963) work shows that bureaucratic characteristics are not all blended together. Some bureaucracies place a greater emphasis on, for example, technical qualifications, rather than rule following. Peter Blau and Richard Scott's (1963) research also suggests that the characteristics of a bureaucracy do not penetrate organizations the same way. Some, such as religious organizations, have goals that counter the unintended negative consequences of efficiency, specialization, and depersonalization. Amitai Etzioni's (1961) analysis of motivational variation relates to this point. It argues that three basic types of motive exist in bureaucracies: love, fear, and money. For example, nuns in a convent might submit to organizational discipline for the love of God. A prisoner in a penitentiary might submit to the discipline of the chain gang in fear of the warden. An industrial worker might submit to the discipline of production because of profit goals. Jerald Hage's (1965) study of organizations shows that the more stratified a bureaucracy is, the less job satisfaction exists.

Other interesting developments on bureaucracy involve a line of thought known as "new institutionalism," which argues that much of contemporary bureaucracy is ceremonial. John Meyer and Brian Rowan's (1991) work indicates that bureaucracies no longer take on Weber's ideal form and people take the conception of a bureaucracy for granted. Instead of having the characteristics of a bureaucracy, organizations now spend more time trying to create an image of what a bureaucracy is supposed to be. So, when external agencies check on an organization to see if it meets certain requirements, the organization being checked focuses on written rules and credentials to maintain certification. In relation to Erving Goffman's (1959) work, this version of new institutionalism implies organizations seek to maintain a bureaucratic façade in order to retain legitimacy (for more on this with respect to nursing homes see Ulsperger and Paul 2002).

Roger Friedland and Robert Alford's (1991) work contends "institutional logics" dominate organizations. These ways of thinking drive the goals of the organization, but also shape the thoughts of people by telling them how to order reality and make sense of the world. Five types of logic exist in U.S. organizations. They are democracy, the nuclear family, Christian religion, the capitalist market, and the bureaucratic state. Democratic logic focuses on communal participation and state control over human activity. Nuclear family logic concerns unconditional loyalty. Religious logic provides a moral frame of reference based on the supernatural. Capitalist logic focuses on accumulation and revenue generation. Bureaucratic logic emphasizes rationality and regulation. The existence of five logics dispels the traditional view that all organizations operate with an emphasis on bureaucratic traits. As you will find later in this book, nursing home bureaucracies can, in fact, have competing logics that influence the way employees think and behave. These have the ability to facilitate and hinder maltreatment of residents.

Writings such as James Coleman's (1985) explain that bureaucratic environments can encourage deviance. As mentioned earlier in this chapter, informal norms can run against the formal norms of the bureaucracy. They can also contradict widespread social values. However, people can normalize themselves to deviant actions in bureaucratic settings. When this occurs, they no longer see the illegal activity in a negative light. For example, consider a situation where a nurse aide sees other aides ritualistically verbally abuse residents day after day. If the aide continues working for the facility, he or she might start to see such deviant behavior as acceptable (also see Simon 1985).

Diane Vaughan's (1992, 1999) work makes a similar argument. It indicates deviance in bureaucracies is the result of routine nonconformity, which leads to mistakes, misconduct, and disasters. Mistakes occur due to a lack of communication between hierarchical levels. In nursing homes, consider problems that might result from poor communication between nurses and administrators. Misconduct can be prompted when competition exists with other organizations. Think of two nursing homes owned by the same corporation in the same area. Administrators might bend the rules when competing with each other to turn higher profits, or staff might lie to state inspectors to lower infraction rates. Disasters take place because of an overload of bureaucratic regulations. When too many guidelines for behavior exist, workers drift away from formal rules toward practical procedures that actually work in the bureaucratic context. For example, a nursing home employee might have to bathe residents with physical limitations, but due to his or her demands to carry out other rule-related tasks, letting the residents bathe themselves seems more practical. In addition, because the employee has never had problems when letting residents with physical problems bathe themselves, that employee reasons that nothing bad will happen (also see Rabe and Ermann 1995; Lee and Ermann 1999).

Another recent, intriguing twist on bureaucracy involves George Ritzer's (2008a) work. He proposes that the fast-food industry, specifically McDonald's, fine-tuned bureaucratic processes. Other organizations picked up on these fast-food interaction patterns to create the "McDonaldization" of America. Building on the notion of bureaucracies, this theory indicates that the typical fast-food restaurant focuses on efficiency, calculability, predictability, and control through nonhuman technology. From a bureaucratic standpoint efficiency requires optimizing the means that lead to an organizational end. For fast-food, think of the objective of providing large numbers of people with a specific product. Calculability is a focus on counting things. For example, McDonald's points out that they have sold billions of burgers and that they serve large amounts of food for small prices. Predictability allows the ability to know outcomes in advance. When you enter a McDonald's, there are no surprises. The one you visit in Tulsa, OK, is likely to look like one you visit in Anchorage, AK. The burgers you get at both places will taste nearly, if not exactly, the same. Control through nonhuman technology is self-explanatory. At McDonald's, technology controls customer actions while waiting for food, both inside the facility and outside in the drive-through line. It also measures the precise amount of ingredients that go into, for example, beverage containers.

Ritzer's writing implies that McDonaldized organizations, like any bureaucracy, can be dysfunctional (Bryman 2005). Have you ever been to McDonald's and thought that people should call it slow food instead of fast food? Have you ever gotten down the road after going through a drive-through and found out you had a Filet-O-Fish instead of a Big Mac? In this book, we argue that nursing homes are highly bureaucratized. However, we think an interesting thing to keep in the back of your mind as you read through the rest of this book is whether the long-term care industry has McDonaldized nursing homes.

Understanding Rituals

Rituals are formal and informal acts with symbolic significance. They involve repeated behaviors that create a balance between individuals and the world. If we did not engage in them on a daily basis, we would feel continuously disoriented—what sociologists call anomie. Some people confuse ritual with routine. For example, you might comment that having a cup of coffee after waking up is your morning ritual (Terrin 2007; Thomassen 2006). Is it? If done enough, getting a cup out of the dishwasher, starting the coffee maker, pouring the beverage, and flavoring it with just the right amount of sugar becomes routine because it happens frequently. It is a ritual only if those processes and your identification with them carry symbolic weight. Do people identify you with coffee? Are you the family's big coffee drinker? Do you wrap your identity up in coffee drinking? Do people at work identify you with it? If so, it really is a ritual.

Some people argue that when you observe a ritual, you are observing social rules in action. When you participate in a ritual, you are conforming to social structure. In other words, rituals have the ability to reinforce the status quo and contribute to the maintenance of power structures (Terrin 2007). Steven Lukes's (1975) and Maurice Bloch's (1989) writings argue that people in power can intentionally promote certain rituals to maintain their domination. Keep in mind, though, that not all people mindlessly follow ritual patterns (Cohen 1993). Even within nursing home environments, residents will resist rituals that place them in objectified, subordinate positions with their own rituals (a point we discuss later in the book).

Ritual Studies

We do not want to devote an excessive amount of attention to the entire history of ritual studies. Work dedicated to that already exists (see Bell 1992). We just want to give you a sample of information on some of the research.

Emile Durkheim ([1912] 1965) was one of the first sociologists to study rituals. His work discusses religious rituals and social unity. When people participate in religious activities, their selfishness dissolves. Religious rituals also reflect and reinforce social values and norms. After Durkheim, secular rituals such as national ceremonies and holidays became a focus of study. For example, Edward Shils and Michael Young's (1953) work analyzes the British Coronation. W. Lloyd Warner's (1959) research supports the notion that Memorial Day is a ritualistic form of community unity. Christmas, Thanksgiving, and the Fourth of July perform similar functions (Warner 1962; Etzioni 2000). And Robert Bellah's (1968) work contends that political speeches have themes that relate to religion to give them a higher level of social legitimacy and to invoke national solidarity.

Studies of legal rituals are interesting. The work of Thurman Arnold (1935) and Jerome Frank (1936) indicates that appellate court decisions act as verifications of legal order. Harold Garfinkel's (1956) findings show trial rituals exist to degrade offenders and promote state authority. Peter Manning's (1977) research shows that police rituals generate a myth that the cops actually control crime, when in reality they tend to just react to it. Life course rituals are equally intriguing. Arnold van Gennep's ([1908] 1960) work connects rites of passage of birth, puberty, procreation, aging, and death to biological changes. Building on the ritual-biology link, Eugene D'Aquili and Andrew Newberg's (1999) work actually links participation in rituals to variation in brainwave activity and blood flow. Durkheim's ([1912] 1965) work supports this idea with a discussion of how religious rituals trigger emotional states in which individuals feel lifted out of themselves. Rituals create a smooth transition to new roles when biology deems them necessary (see Nadel 1954; Turner 1969). Consider a retirement party. Physically a person may no longer be able to work. Socially, speeches, plaques, and a farewell toast give a symbolic end to what is sometimes a necessary biological withdrawal from employment (Savishinsky 1995).

Erving Goffman's (1959) work on everyday life rituals is some of the most fascinating. It places an emphasis on life as rituals of drama. Using a theatrical analogy, he suggests that with everyday rituals, we attempt to generate good impressions of ourselves to others. Think about any first date you have had. You probably attempted to put on a favorable show. You probably bathed, shaved, and applied a nice fragrance somewhere apart from the other person (the backstage). You put on the right costume (clothes). You might have even prepared for the evening by planning out what to talk about (a script). You did all of this to put on a great performance for the other person (your audience).

Goffman's (1961) writings also concern rituals in organizations. They involve unspoken rules on interaction. His research on one organization finds that employees exchange salutations when they pass each other, but the length depends on the time between the last salutation and estimated time before the next. While sitting at lunch tables, staff members give a brief smile when eye contact happens with others because anything less represents a lack of respect. These taken-for-granted actions seem meaningless on the surface, but Goffman's work opens our eyes to how important they are when considering their symbolism.

Goffman's (1967) later work integrates the term "interaction rituals." These happen in everyday encounters. They are unconscious codes people use to acknowledge a shared reality. They build our confidence in social relationships. They also provide us with the ability to confirm our social status and role expectations. In essence, Goffman argues that the idea of rituals Durkheim applied to religion applies to rituals in nearly all face-to-face interactions. Rituals create stability and cohesion. However, social order is not something that exists outside of us. It is something that we achieve through interaction. Overall, it is the situation and not the person that is of importance.

Goffman's writings also discuss "face-work." This is what most of us refer to as "saving face" after an embarrassing situation. When embarrassed, we use rituals to repair our image. This can include using a face of avoidance, repair, or aggression. Consider a co-worker making fun of you in front of others at the office. With avoidance rituals, you might simply dodge the person who embarrassed you until the impact of his or her comment passes. In terms of face repair, you might talk to the person in front of others in a cordial way to create the impression that you blew off the comment made previously. With an aggressive face, you might engage in open conflict with the person to reestablish your damaged status (1967). These rituals are critical to the way you view yourself and also to how others view you.

Randall Collins (2004) builds on Goffman with his idea of interaction ritual chains. His work implies that Goffman was on the right track, but he failed to acknowledge the connection of interaction rituals. With interaction ritual chains, society socializes people to have an intellectual toolkit of rituals with symbolic meaning. People communicate successfully with others using those same rituals and symbols, and feelings of membership and certain amounts of emotional energy emerge as a result. When interaction rituals fail, negative energy occurs. People gravitate toward situations where they know others communicate through the same rituals and situations where they think successful interaction is likely in order to get the biggest emotional payoff.

An interesting example of this process involves firefighters. A key aspect of firefighting is the identity that goes along with it, but also specific types of human interaction for people within the profession. In other words, firefighters create unity through shared symbols and practices identified with firefighting (such as logos with axes and wearing helmets) but also through the interactive process of fighting fires with others. Interestingly, the emotion gained from firefighting creates a feeling of community that lessens the fear most people would feel when fighting a fire. The emotional energy gained from hanging out with other firefighters sometimes causes firefighters to spend leisure time at the station instead of at home (Collins 2004).

Bureaucracy as Ritual

In this book, we use the term organizational culture. It is important to explain what this is and how it relates to rituals. According to the work of social psychologist Joanne Martin, organizational culture involves "stories, humor, jargon, physical arrangements, and formal structures and policies, as well as informal norms and practices" (2002: 55). Her writings emphasize that a key part of all of these components involves rituals. We follow this line of thought believing that rituals are the glue that holds bureaucracies together. While focusing on rituals, this book reviews multiple aspects of nursing homes as organizations to analyze bureaucracy and resident maltreatment. Organizational culture is both shared and unique (Martin 2002). For example, nursing homes as bureaucracies can share qualities with other bureaucracies such as hospitals. At the same time, when you read about nursing home culture in this book, specifically the bureaucratic aspects of it, you might find similarities relating to other organizations, such as prisons.

Few considered rituals to be an important part of organizational culture before the 1980s (for exceptions see Clark 1972; Pettigrew 1979; Selznick 1957). However, throughout the 1980s, people like Michael Rosen (1985) and Harrison Trice and Janice Beyer (1993) started using Goffman's dramaturgical ideas to analyze organizations. When they did, a focus on rituals could not help but break through. They helped lead to the new institutionalism perspective found in Walter Powell and Paul DiMaggio's (1991) collected work on new institutionalism, some of which we discussed earlier.

Structural Ritualization Theory

To study the organizational culture of nursing homes, we follow the tradition of ritual studies previously discussed while acknowledging the idea of bureaucracy as ritual. More precisely, we use a new perspective known as *structural ritualization theory* (SRT), which concentrates on the role of rituals in social life (Knottnerus 1997, 2005, 2009, 2010). The theory is used to analyze, among other things, nursing home resident narratives, employee slang, the physical layout of facilities, administrative structures, formal rules, and informal norms.[1]

As with other perspectives, SRT assumes ritualization involves interaction sequences that occur in multiple contexts including both secular and sacred settings. However, it provides a more dynamic view of rituals due to its systematic focus on ritual action, which it identifies as *ritualized symbolic practices* (RSPs). The theory argues that four factors are essential to the occurrence of RSPs and their ability to influence structural reproduction, a term that refers to the replication or recreation of RSPs and the organization of relationships within and among groups. These factors are *repetitiveness*, *salience*, *homologousness*, and *resources*.

Repetitiveness involves the "relative frequency with which a RSP is performed" (Knottnerus 1997: 262). The idea here is that the repetition of RSPs varies. Great differences may exist in the degree to which RSPs occur in different social settings or domains of interaction. For example, in one area within an organization such as a cafeteria, actors may never engage in a specific RSP. In another, such as a boss's office, people may repeatedly engage in it. Salience involves the "degree to which a RSP is perceived to be central to an act, action sequence, or bundle of interrelated acts" (Knottnerus 1997: 262). This involves the prominence of an RSP, which too can vary. In other words, actors' perceptions of ritualized practices can differ in the extent to which they stand out. Homologousness implies a "degree of perceived similarity among different RSPs" (Knottnerus 1997: 263). It is possible that different RSPs exist in a social setting. However, they may or may not be similar in meaning and form. The more they are alike, the more likely they strengthen each other. This enhances the impact of RSPs. Finally, resources are "materials needed to engage in RSPs and that are available to actors" (Knottnerus 1997: 264). The greater the availability of resources, the more likely an individual will participate in an RSP. Resources include nonhuman materials such as money, time, clothes or uniforms, and physical items (e.g., musical instruments, furniture, buildings). They also include human traits such as intellectual capacity, interaction skills, physical strength, and cognitive abilities.

Rank is another important concept in the theory. It involves "the relative standing of a RSP in terms of its dominance" or importance (Knottnerus 1997: 266). According to the theory, rank is a function of repetitiveness, salience, homologousness, and resources. An RSP ranks high if it is repeated often, is quite visible, is similar to other RSPs, and people have the resources to take part in it. RSPs with a high rank are more likely to influence the way people think and act and lead to the reproduction of ritualized behaviors and relationships.

Subsequent chapters examine daily, taken-for-granted RSPs of bureaucracy that facilitate RSPs of emotional, physical, and verbal maltreatment of nursing home residents. Integrating personal stories from residents, family members, and employees of nursing homes, we assess the rank of RSPs of bureaucracy and maltreatment in nursing homes using measures of repetitiveness and salience. However, before we turn to the analysis of RSPs of bureaucracy and resident neglect and abuse, it is important to understand how one of the major social trends of our time, bureaucracy, influenced the development of nursing homes.

Note

1. For additional research utilizing the theory, see Knottnerus 1999, 2002; Knottnerus and Van de Poel-Knottnerus 1999; Van de Poel-Knottnerus and Knottnerus 2002; Sell, Knottnerus, Ellison, and Mundt 2000; Edwards and Knottnerus 2007, 2010; Knottnerus and Berry 2002; Knottnerus and LoConto 2003; Knottnerus, Monk, and Jones 1999; Knottnerus, Ulsperger, Cummins, and Osteen 2006; Minton and Knottnerus 2008; Mitra and Knottnerus 2004, 2008; Sarabia and Knottnerus 2009; Thornburg, Knottnerus, and Webb 2007, 2008; Ulsperger and Knottnerus 2007, 2008a, 2008b, 2009a, 2009b; Varner and Knottnerus 2002; Wu and Knottnerus 2005, 2007.

CHAPTER 3
A HISTORY OF NURSING HOMES

The law is unfair.... It is like a cure for the crime
that's much greater than the crime.
  David Banks, Former Beverly Enterprises CEO

Jan Richards's father was in a Beverly Health and Rehabilitation
nursing home in Frankfort, KY. In the early part of March 2002, he
complained to staff about constipation issues. One employee gave
him some milk of magnesia, but his stomach remained swollen and
bloated. He had been vomiting for days. By noon, he started yelling
for a nurse to help him and pleading that he did not want to die.
According to his family, no one was at the nurses' station to hear
his cries. He died soon after (Williamson 2006; Yetter 2006).

A few weeks later, Jan was in church, and a man who worked
for the city driving nursing home residents around town spoke
to her. He told her that it was a shame her father had to suffer
with little done by the employees to help. She was confused. She
thought the facility did a good job caring for him. When she
found out her hard-working father, who had been a farmer and
forklift operator, died pleading for help, she was angry. She, her

brother Phil, and sister Wanda Delaplane, wanted answers, but the nursing home employees were not talking. Delaplane, an assistant attorney general in Kentucky, approached a state agency set up to monitor Kentucky's nursing home care. She found out that when her father died, thirteen employees were working. However, ten were on a work break. That left three staff members to tend to all of the home's one hundred residents. It was no surprise that no one heard Loren Richards's pleas. Though Kentucky had no law at the time dictating a specific staff-resident ratio, Delaplane sued (Billups 2006; Yetter 2006).

According to the attorneys representing the family, the nursing home was clearly negligent and responsible for Loren's death. Employees even falsified documents to cover up their understaffing at the time of the incident. Family attorneys argued that the home cut back on employees merely to raise profits. On the contrary, Beverly attorneys argued Loren received superb care, employees loved him, and he always appeared happy. Moreover, his daughters visited him frequently and would have spoken up or moved him to another home if they thought care in the facility was declining (Williamson 2006).

After the trial, Delaplane stated, "I had to live my dad's death over each day, but it was worth it" (Billups 2006: 98). One Beverly attorney believed the "worth" was all about money for the Richards family, indicating that a once-proposed $159 million settlement was offensive. He went on to say that even a $100,000 settlement would be offensive because the nursing home provided great care. In May 2006, a civil jury returned a $20 million verdict in favor of the Richards family. The nursing home appealed and an out-of-court settlement was reached (Billups 2006; Williamson 2006).

Did nursing home greed lead to the death? Did family greed create an unnecessary civil trial? The answer to these questions is not easy to establish in the litigious society in which we live.

However, we believe there are a few things that people fail to discuss in situations like Loren Richards's. First, how did we end up putting aged loved ones in facilities called nursing homes in the first place? Second, how did greed and profit get tangled up in nursing home life? How did bureaucratic thinking, which can lead to organizational mistakes that could result in death, come to saturate our nursing homes? Finally, as former Beverly Enterprises CEO David Banks argued in a *Healthweek* interview (Mayer 1989), is nursing home law unfair? Does it actually promote long-term care problems?

Elder Care in Early American History

Some people view the nursing home industry as an outgrowth of Medicare and Medicaid. We believe its roots are older and more complex. We see the contemporary nursing home as an extension of early colonial life in the 1700s. Then, public policy followed the tradition of English poor laws. They left the care of elderly in the hands of community governments. For the aged in America, this meant the only form of public support was institutional. Society left the responsibility of caring for the destitute aged to poor farms.

Colonial Poor Farms

By lumping all of the unwanted of society into one group, poor farms, also known as almshouses, managed the care of the poor, sick, mentally ill, and lawbreakers. The first poor farms in the United States appeared in Boston, Philadelphia, and New York. They held as many as 100,000 elderly Americans (Hawes and Phillips 1986; Vladeck 1980).

Many poor farms were actually in homes known as poor houses. The community would build or acquire homes for sale and change them to meet the needs of impoverished occupants. In order to deter poverty and crime, the conditions in poor houses were intentionally left substandard, so people would avoid them at all costs. Usually, people did not place the elderly in a poor house unless they had very little personal or family support. There was no stigma attached to being old, frail, and without resources. Communities, typically with a strong religious base, supported the process of aging. They viewed it as a virtue. In fact, religious organizations would often run poor houses (Giacalone 2001).

Care for the aged in poor houses had a religious tone, but also a family one. Administrators viewed the aged as extended family, and the social structure of the facilities was informal. Few employees existed because able-bodied residents carried out most of the chores. Though people did not look down on the old-poor, few attempts to improve social conditions occurred (Lidz, Fischer, and Arnold 1992).

Negative Images of the Elderly in the 1800s

In 1828, Andrew Jackson became the first president born poor, and many of his policies focused on cures for various aspects of poverty. Dependency was no longer a sore that religious groups placed a bandage over. It was a secular problem that was repairable with the appropriate reforms. Institutions for the destitute increased in number, while a movement started to separate the unwanted of society into different groups. Specific facilities emerged to house orphans, criminals, and the aged. Being more bureaucratic in nature, these new institutions used systematic rules and routines, and focused on discipline (Lidz, Fischer, and Arnold 1992; Wallbank et al. 1992).

Problems for the poor and old continued. As the 1800s un-folded, they quickly lost their Jacksonian status as equal members of society. People viewed the destitute old as responsible for their own difficulties. The elderly lost prestige as younger citizens started believing that inferior moral habits were the cause of illness and dependency in old age. Attitudes shifted against government-supported institutions for the elderly. The wealthy did establish quality old-age homes that provided medical assistance to people with the proper social backgrounds. However, substandard care continued for those without means (Achenbaum 1978; Cole 1987; Giacalone 2001).

The Birth of the Contemporary Nursing Home

The population of the United States shot up in the early twentieth century. In addition, the Industrial Revolution resulted in more people living in urban areas. Elevated immigration created an ample amount of conflict between social groups. In order to control a select category of immigrants and homeless juveniles, society started placing even more people in institutions. Policy makers promoted this agenda in the name of social order and under the veil of criminal justice. Interestingly, many Americans who were eager to institutionalize immigrants and homeless juveniles did not want to continue to stigmatize the aged in the same way. The move to create independence for the aged with public pensions reflects this attitude (Vold, Bernard, and Snipes 2002; Vladeck 1980).

The Fraternal Order of the Eagles was one of the first groups to fight for pensions. They claimed that caring for the aged was a social responsibility. By 1923, their efforts led to pensions for the elderly in Pennsylvania, Montana, and Nevada. Other states adopted similar plans (Achenbaum 1978). The California "ham and eggs" group also influenced pension development. The label "ham and eggs" emerged when a speaker addressing campaign workers promised that their group would be as familiar as ham and eggs to California voters. Their plan proposed weekly payments of $25 to every jobless citizen over the age of 50. Fraud-related problems led to the disintegration of the movement (Mitchell 2000; Putnam 1970). Pension plans came under fire in the 1930s. One of these was the Townsend Plan, which called for providing $200 per month to those 60 years or older. It gained positive publicity, but soon drifted into oblivion (Powell, Branco, and Williamson 1996).

The federal government gave in to the call to provide support for the poor-old in the New Deal era with the 1935 Social Security Act. Politicians labeled the first title of the act Old Age Assistance (OAA). The program provided federal payments of no more than $30 to recipients. You had to meet state-defined requirements to get a payment. States would then match the federal payment. OAA was need-based, so policy makers designed it to provide income to the elderly who did not get full benefits from old-age insurance, another part of the act. OAA did allow recipients to use the funds as they pleased. Because of scandals and criticisms involving poor farms, regulations prohibited the institutionalized elderly in public facilities from receiving payments. However, private pay homes could receive payments. This is the time when what we now identify as nursing homes emerged. In 1939, before people took full advantage of OAA, only 1,200 nursing homes existed. By 1963, the number increased to 12,800 (Hawes and Phillips 1986).

When the contemporary nursing home first emerged, un-employed nurses operated them in their houses. It was a way of creating extra income, especially as the country recovered from the Great Depression. The care in many of these facilities seemed suitable, but objections about conditions quickly spread. Stories of physical and financial abuse leaked to the public. However, high demand persuaded politicians to ignore calls for improvements (Lidz, Fischer, and Arnold 1992).

OAA Funding and Elder Care Capitalism

In the 1940s, women entered the formal workforce in numbers larger than ever. With many working-age men in the service, female labor became a necessity as t.he United States ramped up the production of wartime materials used during World War II. Occupied by employment out of the household, some of these women turned over the care of aged loved ones to institutions such as nursing homes. Adding to the growth of nursing homes, OAA continued to feed the for-profit industry in the 1940s as the nature of nursing homes changed. They became larger and more medically oriented. As facilities no longer remained family-type environments, residents came to expect formal care focused on rules, larger staffs with a hierarchical structure, and an orientation to medical services. Facilities started looking less like homes and more like hospitals. Laws passed to help expand the hospital industry during this time also greatly influenced nursing home growth (Vladeck 1980).

Consider the Hill-Burton Act (HBA) of 1946. It initially provided funding for hospital construction, but soon funded the construction of nonprofit nursing homes. Around this time, amendments to the Social Security Act allowed people to use their OAA money on services provided by nonprofit and for-profit facilities. State, religious, and fraternal organizations started building more nursing homes than ever before. On the surface, it appeared nonprofit homes reaped the most benefit. This, however, was not the case. Changes in OAA funding and government loans for nursing home construction attracted a plethora of entrepreneurs. Though they were out of the loop when it came to construction funds under the HBA, they discovered that loans through the Small Business Administration and Federal Housing Act covered their construction and supply costs. It was obvious that a capitalist logic was building in the nursing home industry as the shift from welfare to health care continued (Lidz, Fischer, and Arnold 1992).

OAA funding started going to institutions, and people receiving it were no longer directly involved with payments. The for-profit nursing home industry began to lobby for OAA funding increases and to dissuade politicians from closely monitoring care (Hawes and Phillips 1986). The American Association of Nursing Homes emerged in 1949 as the leading lobby group for for-profit nursing home owners. It merged with the National Association of Registered Nursing Homes in 1956 and was renamed the American Nursing Home Administration. It is now the American Health Care Association. It has for-profit and nonprofit members. The branch exclusively devoted to for-profit owners is the Alliance for Quality Nursing Home Care (AHCA 2008; Williams 1999). Nonprofit nursing homes developed their own exclusive lobby group in 1961. It currently goes by the name the American Association of Homes and Services for the Aging (AAHSA 2008; Giacalone 2001).

We believe it is worth noting that many of the names connected to the for-profit industry during the heyday of OAA funding used shady practices to generate revenue. Sources indicate some even had ties to the Mafia (see Mendelson 1974). Regardless, lobby groups convinced policy makers to pump more money into the industry, and national expenditures increased substantially. Money made from nursing homes reached $33 million in 1940, $187 million in 1950, and $1.3 billion by 1965 (Giacalone 2001). They paid only 10 percent of expenses, but by the 1960s, it was 22 percent. More nursing homes than ever existed, and with the U.S. General Accounting Office reporting a nursing home bed shortage, more were on the way (Hawes and Phillips 1986).

Industry Expansion through Medicare and Medicaid

The 1960s began with the Kerr-Mills Act, also known as the Hospital Survey and Construction Act. It replaced OAA with Medical Assistance for the Aged (MAA) and allowed states to control the criteria for government assistance. It also removed the federal responsibility to match state funds. By 1965, MAA money provided support for more than half of nursing home residents (Lidz, Fischer, and Arnold 1992). The establishment of MAA was important, but the 1965 amendments to the Social Security Act continue to be the most relevant policies concerning elder care because they implemented Medicare and Medicaid (Giacalone 2001).

Medicare

Medicare is a government program that provides the primary source of health insurance for people 65 and older. The designers of the program created it for hospitals, but inflated costs made low-priced alternatives to hospital care attractive. Later amendments made the use of extended-care facilities, such as nursing homes, acceptable. Medicare funds around 10 percent of nursing home costs (Hawes and Phillips 1986; Kahana 2000).

Part A of Medicare, known as hospital insurance, pays for in-patient acute care in hospitals and some skilled nursing services. It covers things such as intravenous feeding, treatment of skin disorders, speech, and occupational therapy. Part B pays for physician fees, some aspects of home care, and medical supplies (other parts exist that exclusively concern Medicare HMO and prescription drugs). If your aged loved one receives Part A benefits through a nursing home, be careful to observe what the facility says it will or will not cover. For example, some nursing homes say Part A will not cover therapy unless an improvement in the resident's condition occurs. However, if the therapy helps the resident maintain his or her condition, it might. Also, remember that you do not have to get a multitude of services to qualify. Just one is sufficient. Nursing homes have a lot of discretion in initially deciding if someone is qualified for Part A coverage. In turn, you should emphasize to the facility staff, and the resident's doctor, that your aged loved one needs *skilled services*. Medicare will only cover the variety of services discussed previously if they carry that moniker. If a facility determines that a resident should no longer receive skilled services through this program, it must provide a written notice. If you disagree, you can appeal through the Centers for Medicare and Medicaid Services. If you do, the nursing home cannot charge you for services while the dispute is considered.

The use of Medicare is limited. It pays for the first twenty-one days of a nursing home stay, and that is only after a minimum three-night hospital stay. Afterward, days twenty-one to one hundred, residents must pay a little more than $100 per day for Medicare to pick up the rest. After one hundred days, coverage is over (Carlson and Hsiao 2006). Currently, with a daily rate around $200, many elderly residents do not have the extra funds to cover a longer stay and end up depleting their savings. Thirty percent of elderly residents are in poverty within three months of nursing home admission (MetLife 2006; Rosen and Wilbur 1992). That impoverishment leads to Medicaid eligibility.

Medicaid

Medicaid is a decentralized program operating between the federal and state level that provides sustained medical services to poor people. If an elderly person in a nursing home qualifies for Medicaid, it will cover room, board, and routine nursing services. It will also cover therapy, non-prescription drugs, doctor's visits, optometry services, hearing aids, prosthetics, and ambulance service (and a variety of other things excluding commodities such as clothing). Medicaid pays for 60 percent of nursing home expenses (Giacalone 2001).

Nursing home Medicaid issues vary depending on marriage status. If a person is not married, 65 and older or disabled, and does not have resources typically exceeding $2,000, then they are eligible. A home is not a resource if the resident plans to return to it. Income is not relevant in determining eligibility, but after a person is determined eligible, income will determine how much he or she pays toward care and how much Medicaid will cover. If someone is just over the cap for eligibility, it is possible to put a small portion of income into a trust to obtain coverage. Moreover, if a person is unmarried, it is possible to keep a portion of monthly income for personal needs. This amount varies from state to state from between $30 and $90 (Carlson and Hsiao 2006).

In the past, if a person was married, getting Medicaid coverage was not possible unless the spouse depleted all of the couple's resources to get below the previously discussed eligibility limit, but that has changed. Now, a spouse can have 50 percent of the couple's available resources at the time of nursing home entry. Moving resources from one spouse to the other does not affect eligibility; however, after a person is eligible, an increased amount of resources for the at-home spouse will not disqualify the nursing home resident. Be careful if you plan to shift assets to people other than a spouse. Some families try to give away resources for "temporary keeping" in order to gain Medicaid eligibility. However, the program will consider any resources given away during the five years prior to applying (Carlson and Hsiao 2006).

After the passage of Medicare and Medicaid legislation in 1965, nursing home growth exploded. Nearly ten years after approval of the programs, the number of nursing home beds in the United

States had increased to more than 1 million and the number of facilities reached slightly more than 15,700. With more people entering homes in the late 1960s and 1970s, the government needed to attract providers, so they adopted two policies: increased reimbursement rates and decreased concern with regulation (Hawes and Phillips 1986).

Medicare adopted a cost-based reimbursement policy grounded in reported expenditures. There were no ceilings on reimbursements. The government ignored variations between providers. In addition, it provided income to for-profit owners on their net invested equity in a facility. In other words, owners did not have to worry about meeting their mortgage in the first few years of operation. The government would cover it. This allowed facilities a guaranteed profit (Shulman and Galanter 1976; Vladeck 1980).

In terms of regulations, the government did require Medicare- and Medicaid-funded homes to meet certain requirements to receive funds. The same policy exists today. States have government workers survey nursing homes to make sure they meet minimum requirements. In the early stages of funding, facilities participating had to provide twenty-four-hour nursing services, have a registered nurse, and rotate the nurse on duty each shift. Requirements also included (and still do) areas of medical supervision, pharmacy services, fire safety, diet, and sanitation programs (Giacalone 2001).

Following the passage of the Social Security Act of 1965, policy makers estimated that few nursing homes could meet the minimum standards. Out of the first 6,000 institutions that applied for Medicare and Medicaid funds, only 10 percent were eligible (Lidz, Fischer, and Arnold 1992). Legislation known as the Moss Amendments provided laws to improve nursing home standards, but the government quickly decided to give facilities funds if they were in *substantial compliance*, rather than full compliance. When a state survey agency found violations, nursing homes had only to present them with a plan for corrections and nothing else. This made it easy for owners seeking profit to cut operating costs. For-profit owners believed such a move could lead to an increased number of infractions, but the only result would be a minor revision of their plan of operation. In conjunction with this change, the federal government passed the Miller Amendment in 1971. It established a new classification system for nursing homes. Nursing homes could be intermediate-care facilities. The law did not require these facilities to have the same amount of resources, such as skilled nursing staff, that traditional facilities had in place. As a result, people became increasingly concerned with the quality of nursing home care (Giacalone 2001; Hawes and Phillips 1986).

The Emergence of Scandal

Although complaints about nursing home conditions existed in the 1960s, nursing home care as a social problem came to the forefront in the 1970s. Scandals involving low-quality care, Medicaid and Medicare fraud, and deviant political influence swept the country. The most infamous series of scandals happened in 1975. New York residents called that year the "Year of the Investigations." The state shut down sixty-three nursing homes that did not comply with federal standards. Officials removed 1,000 beds from over-crowded facilities and established a nursing home abuse hotline, which received more than 1,500 claims of resident maltreatment. The state had to hire extra attorneys because of all of the nursing home prosecutions. A special commission indicted Vice President Nelson Rockefeller, the former governor of New York, and he testified in a televised hearing on his responsibility in the debacle (Hess 1976a, 1976b).

Problems didn't occur just in New York. Policy makers, business owners, and caregivers from all across the country also came under fire. The New York situation was just a small sample of the emerging elder care catastrophe. It was not unusual to find nursing homes serving green meat, residents drowning in bathtubs, and people lying in their own excrement (Vladeck 1980).

One investigation, spearheaded by Ralph Nader, used students from a school in Connecticut working undercover in nursing homes to provide first-hand reports of horrors (Townsend 1971). For-profit facilities gained a reputation for promoting inferior care. It was during this time that research on the differences between for-profit and nonprofit facilities surfaced (see Chapter 1). Regardless of public sentiment and empirical studies, things did not get much better.

Chain Domination and Reform Demands

As the age wave reached the late 1970s and early 1980s, the demand for nursing homes continued despite a decade of turmoil. The Boren Amendment of the Omnibus Reconciliation Act of 1980 mandated that nursing home rates be reasonable. Even so, facilities were charging more while poor care continued. The cost of care soon reached an unprecedented level. The average annual expenditure on one resident went from $5,100 in 1970 to $23,300 by 1985 (Giacalone 2001).

Fewer Homes, More Beds

With respect to federal regulations, states started focusing more on rule violations. Many went beyond federal standards to impose standards of their own. Their intention was good; however, the strict standards put smaller facilities out of business because they could not logistically meet new requirements. Larger for-profit nursing homes, usually part of chains, gained momentum. For them, the regulations of the mid-1980s were not a problem. They met requirements for new standards as they constructed new facilities while smaller homes faded away. This explains why the number of nursing homes peaked in the United States at 19,000 in 1985, but the number of nursing home beds continued to grow. Legal demands also created problems for smaller homes. They promoted a need for specialization. With laws for activities, food, rehabilitation, and the preservation of resident records, facilities needed specific departments to address these individual areas. Certification for certain workers became a requirement. Nursing home care became increasingly bureaucratic and complex (Johnson and Grant 1985; National Center for Health Statistics 2006).

Around this time, policy makers introduced a modified reimbursement system to replace the flat-rate system that let nursing home owners self-report costs and receive full reimbursements. Before the introduction of modified reimbursements, owners operated satellite services. These businesses would provide food and medical equipment for their own facility and then overcharge themselves to maximize profits. This gave them more capital, which in turn allowed them to build more facilities. By 1983, most states switched to a system that put a cap on refund requests. Many now estimate the cost of services before they provide them. In essence, government money started coming in on the front end of the process (Giacalone 2001).

This still played to the advantage of for-profit facilities. Chains that expanded under the old system had the resources to find loopholes in the prepay provisions. They hired financial experts who had the ability to manipulate the new system. The smaller facilities, which were more familiar with the flat-rate policy, did not understand the stock-swaps, intercompany loans, and lease-back arrangements that helped the bigger facilities to dominate (Giacalone 2001; Hawes and Phillips 1986). Again, a policy designed to put larger, for-profit facilities on their toes contributed to their growth. New laws ironically seemed to be creating more problems.

The Omnibus Budget Reconciliation Act of 1987

The Institute of Medicine came out with a scathing report on nursing homes in 1985. Unlike with previous reports, this one seemed to matter. It helped lead to the Omnibus Budget Reconciliation Act of 1987 (OBRA), also known as the Nursing Home Reform Act. Policy makers designed OBRA to decrease levels of inept care, and it continues to have a large effect on facilities. Its provisions remove divisions between an SNF and an ICF. Agencies now typically refer to all nursing homes as nursing facilities (NFs). In addition, nursing homes that receive public funding now must meet new, more demanding standards. These standards include an emphasis on quality-of-life issues, with a push to help residents maintain and improve ADLs. They also focus on nursing homes creating personal, individualized plans of care for each resident; allowing residents to choose personal physicians; and facilitating the creation of family and resident councils. Other provisions involve points on staff education, employee staffing levels, and visitor rights (Filinson 1995; Giacalone 2001).

With respect to maltreatment, OBRA established the formal right for residents to be free from threats or abuse. This includes mental and physical abuse relating to corporal punishment, drugs, or physical restraints to control residents, as well as involuntary isolation. OBRA also makes results from state surveys available to family members and residents, which allows them to formally see which areas of care their facility does not adequately provide

(Mooney and Greenway 1996). After establishment of the new guidelines, violations declined and staffing levels increased in nursing homes (Zhang and Grabowski 2004). Analysts imply that the political influence of the for-profit nursing home owners may have had a hand in distorting survey results following OBRA (Harrington and Carrillo 1999).

The Nursing Home Reform Movement

Efforts by organizations like the National Citizens' Coalition for Nursing Home Reform (NCCNHR) played, and continue to play, an important role in the history of nursing homes. The group's creation marks the formal establishment of the nursing home reform movement. NCCNHR appeared in 1975 out of a concern to improve facility conditions. Citizen groups and ombudsman program members met at a National Gray Panthers meeting in Washington, DC, to discuss long-term care. For years the Gray Panthers had been fighting for issues concerning the elderly. The meeting allowed important figures concerned with nursing home issues to come together for one of the first times. Knowing an American Health Care Association meeting was on the way, attendees decided to construct a presentation on nursing home issues.

Elma Holder, NCCNHR founder, feverishly pushed for resident-friendly legislation from the organization's inception. Her efforts helped shape laws that established government-sponsored long-term care ombudsman programs, typically operated through Area Agencies on Aging in every state. Ombudsmen continue to be important resources in the effort to improve nursing home life. NCCNHR membership currently includes more than two hundred groups and 1,000 individuals. The coalition's stated goal is to continue developing strategies to improve the quality of life of residents. It carries out this task by promoting residents' rights.

NCCNHR also calls for minimizing the use of physical and chemical restraints. With respect to fiscal abuse, it advocates liability for all excess spending (NCCNHR 2008; Ulsperger 2002). NCCNHR fought hard for OBRA 1987. Some analysts even credit the act's passage to NCCNHR (Filinson 1995). We encourage you to find out as much as possible about this advocacy group if you have an elderly loved one entering or living in a nursing home. Their web site, www.nccnhr.org, provides a great deal of information for nursing home consumers. In addition, when searching for nursing home information seek out similar local groups that exist in a majority of states.

Recent Congressional Activity

In the wake of OBRA, rumblings of nursing home neglect and abuse fell off in the 1990s. Yet NCCNHR members and others wanted more action in terms of resident quality of life. However, the passage of OBRA created an advocacy hangover. Complaints that policy makers were not doing enough were no longer as powerful as they once had been. In order to thrive, advocacy groups like NCCNHR had to shift the nature of their complaints to more structural issues such as bankruptcy, billing fraud, staff shortages, and staff training (Ulsperger 2002). Nonetheless, in the late 1990s, Congress passed some significant legislation that shook the industry.

The Balanced Budget Act of 1997 repealed some aspects of the Boren Amendment and cut the amount of Medicare nursing homes received. Facilities relied too heavily on Medicare. In addition, many chains built more homes on the expectation of continued Medicare and Medicaid money. Soon, half of the largest nursing home chains filed for bankruptcy, and approximately 1,600 facilities ended up operating under Chapter 11 protection. The Balanced Budget Refinement Act of 1999 attempted to alleviate the problem by restoring funds to the industry. Subsequently, nursing home financing continued to grow; for the 2001 fiscal year, it reached $2.6 billion, up 20 percent from the year before (Pelovitz 2000; Wiener and Stevenson 1998).

In September 2007, a headline appeared in *The New York Times* that looked like it was pulled from the "Year of the Investigations" more than three decades earlier. It read "At Many Homes, More Profit and Less Nursing" (Duhigg 2007). The article described an industry saturated with greedy nursing home owners who typically have their hands in investments like Dunkin' Donuts. It went on to discuss widespread problems such as bedsores infected by feces, staff levels lower than the law allows, and the creation of confusing corporate structures to bypass Medicare–Medicaid reporting rules. On the heels of that article, the House Committee on Energy and Commerce Subcommittee on Oversight and Investigation met in early 2008 to analyze the state of the nursing home industry. Several important players in the field discussed equally interesting and disturbing points. Lewis Morris, the Chief Counsel to the Office of the Inspector General for the Department of Health and Human Services; Luis Navas-Migueloa, Baltimore's long-term care ombudsman; and Kerry Weems, the acting administrator for Centers for Medicare and Medicaid Services (CMS), were among the speakers.

Morris explained that CMS continues to work with state agencies to identify problem nursing homes by using state inspectors who visit facilities once every 15 months. He noted that when facilities do not meet standards, the typical CMS repercussion is to make them provide corrective action plans or impose monetary penalties. The problem with this process is that states do not cite facilities consistently, inspectors fail to have objective guidelines for issuing citations, and state inspector turnover is high. Morris also argued that state inspectors underestimate serious problems in their reports. He stated that only 42 percent of homes fined for infractions pay those fines, and only a fraction of facilities that are supposed to shut down for having residents in serious jeopardy ever close their doors. States are also required to keep nursing aide registration lists indicating whether a person has the appropriate background to work in a nursing home with vulnerable populations. Though most states check their own registries, they seldom check registries from other states. This increases the potential for people with bad intentions to gain employment in long-term care facilities (Morris 2008).

In addition to these troubling points, Morris pointed out some of the current problems with for-profit facilities. Providing some sociological insight related to earlier points in this book, he indicated the increasingly challenging task of proving individual intent in a world dominated by organizations. He explained that corporate nursing homes intentionally create multiple levels of responsibility and power in order to obstruct law enforcement's ability to assign blame when caregiving misconduct occurs. He argued that it is becoming more difficult to determine exactly who is responsible in maltreatment situations. Is it the lower-level employee, the nurse supervisor, the administrator, the CEO, or the stockholders? *The New York Times* article from the previous year noted that 70 percent of lawyers who used to sue nursing homes have stopped doing so because it is too expensive and difficult because of a lack of clear accountability. In one maltreatment case, an attorney had to sue twenty-two different companies and ended up collecting a mere $25,000 (Duhigg 2007).

At the hearing, Navas-Migueloa pointed out that the typical complaints he deals with involve quality-of-life issues, resident-to-resident conflict, and abuse at the hands of nursing staff. Agreeing with Morris, he noted that owners of larger, for-profit facilities hide behind an array of organizational layers. Nursing homes with multiple levels, he argues, are void of human contact and more likely to promote inhumane care (an issue we see existing in nonprofit, highly bureaucratic facilities as well). According to Navas-Migueloa, this organizational detachment leads to poor maintenance, reduced staffing, and pest control problems. On ownership issues and nursing home quality of life, he stated, "If you are looking for the best dining experience, would you rather have dinner in a chain restaurant or one where the chef is the owner?" (Navas-Migueloa 2008: 4).

Navas-Migueloa goes on to tell a story about one facility where the owner was never around. He was visiting with a resident in his room when the strong smell of marijuana hit his nose. He looked out the window and saw employees outside smoking marijuana while taking a break. The resident told him they did it all the time. Navas-Migueloa went to the administrator and questioned the actions of the employees. He knew the facility had security cameras in the area where staff drug use occurred. When he asked the administrator to review the video, the administrator told him that the camera was not recording during the time in question and that he needed to direct any other issues he had to the corporate office. From that point on, the facility was not cooperative with his ombudsman duties (Navas-Migueloa 2008).

Weems started off by stating that 1.5 million Americans are now living in 16,000 nursing homes nationwide, and that more than 3 million Americans depend on nursing homes at some point in any given year. Approximately 1.8 million people receive care paid for through Medicare every year, and Medicare benefits currently stand at $21 billion per year. He went on to state that CMS has a plan of action to improve the quality of nursing homes. That plan currently includes providing nursing home consumers with better information and obtaining more contracts with quality improvement organizations that can go into a nursing home and show them how to run things better. The plan also addresses actively reducing aspects of neglect and abuse, and specifically attempts to reduce the overuse of restraints along with lowering rates of bed sores that result from residents lying immobile for long periods of time. For problems related to chain ownership, he revealed that CMS has the Provider Enrollment Chain and Ownership System (PECOS). The system gathers information on the official owner of a facility, where the nursing home provides services, and whether the facility meets licensing qualifications for CMS payments (Weems 2008).

The acting CMS director also discussed the Special Focus Facility (SFF) Program. The program was actually unveiled a few months earlier, and it caused a small stir when it named more than 100 of the worst nursing homes in the country. It noted that most nursing homes have approximately seven deficiencies when inspected. However, some nursing homes have serious problems, and CMS has to handle them differently. These are SFFs. In February 2008, CMS had identified 131 SFFs. State inspectors visit SFFs twice as often as regular nursing homes (CMS 2008). Weems repeated this riveting information to the Subcommittee on Oversight and Investigations. Committee members did not seem impressed. Members, almost mockingly, restated his point and noted that it meant inspectors visit SFFs only twice a year. Weems indicated that inspectors should visit them more often than that, but CMS does not have the resources needed to do it (Committee on Energy and Commerce 2008).

In early October 2009, the headline "Waves of New Fund Cuts Imperil U.S. Nursing Homes" appeared in newspapers throughout the country and all over the Internet. Associated Press writer Dave Collins reported that the future of nursing homes was bleak as a result of economic recession and funding cuts at every level of government. His article indicated that over the next 10 years, lawmakers plan to cut an estimated $16 billion in nursing home funding. Smaller homes are closing due to budget constraints, and unfortunately more nursing home residents are now ending up in larger, bureaucratic facilities with fewer employees to meet their needs (Collins 2009).

NCCNHR argues that there may be a light at the end of the elder care catastrophe tunnel. The reform-based organization recently released information indicating that the health care legislation passed in early 2010 has the potential to create better nursing homes. Specifically, the bill includes provisions that require the federal government to supply better, and more accurate, information on staffing levels, inspection reports, and sanctions. It provides funding for improved training for people who work for public agencies responsible for investigating nursing home neglect and abuse. It also sets the stage for a national criminal background check program for people employed in the long-term care industry (NCCNHR 2010).

Culture Change

A movement to change the dominant modes of thinking and acting for employees in nursing homes is happening right now. We hope this book will be a part of that movement. People call it *culture change*. It involves ideas such as person-directed care and developing new nursing homes with small, individual dwellings instead of ones based on medical models (see Weiner and Ronch 2003). Chapter 9 discusses culture change in detail. It also explains how our research pertains to culture change.

Chapter 4
Rules over Compassion

Bureaucracy is the art of making the possible
impossible.

Javier Pascual Salcedo

In the hit movie *Wedding Crashers*, the two main characters have
an array of rules they use when showing up at weddings uninvited.
The rules help them reap the benefits of attendance and accomplish
certain goals, such as obtaining free food and, for lack of a better
phrase, physical gratification with the opposite sex (Faber and Fisher
2005). Rules spell out many requirements for everyday interaction,
not just crashing weddings. However, with organizations, it is easy
to see how an overemphasis on rules can create problems the rules
set out to prevent in the first place.

We think quality of life and quality of care are possible in many
nursing homes. In this chapter, we want to illustrate how aspects of
bureaucracy, such as rules, make impossible what we feel should be
possible. Here, and in subsequent chapters on emotional, physical,
and verbal neglect and abuse, we use content analysis results from
our extensive examination of nursing home literature as discussed in

Appendix 1. We also use information from first-hand observations and interviews carried out with nursing home employees.

Negative Aspects of Bureaucracy in Nursing Home Care

Our data indicate that characteristics of bureaucracy dominate nursing home life. In the content analysis portion of this research, more than 2,000 references to RSPs of bureaucracy exist in our sources. As Table 4.1 illustrates, themes focused on staff separation, rules, documentation, and efficiency, all of which we believe inadvertently lead to poor resident care.

Staff Separation and Hierarchy

We define staff separation and hierarchy as any ritualized practice that reinforces dividing lines between staff. With our content analysis, 861 references to staff separation and hierarchy appear, making up 37.8 percent of references. Sources indicate these divisions are often the result of government regulations requiring staff members to have certain educational levels and training certifications. Reflecting what nearly every source indicates, Shield

Table 4.1 Frequencies for Bureaucratic Rituals

Subdivision	Number	Percent
Staff separation and hierarchy	861	37.8
Rules	601	26.4
Documentation	552	24.2
Efficiency	265	11.6
Total	2,279	100.0

(1988: 93) states, "Several implicit hierarchies—medical, administrative, nursing, and social service—operate within the [nursing home] bureaucracy."

Discussions in the sources often involve the importance of work duties in the employment hierarchy. They detail how specific work duties exist exclusively for specific staff members. If an employee assigned a specific duty does not carry out the task, it often goes undone. In one source, for example, residents looked forward to coffee during activity time; coffee was served by the activity director in the activity area. Residents confined to their rooms during this time wanted aides walking by to bring them coffee. Neglecting the desires of residents, aides would not serve coffee because it was not their specifically assigned duty (Kayser-Jones 1981). This indicates that in specific domains of interaction in nursing homes, if a person is not typically required to help a resident in a specific area, the resident will suffer.

Such actions might just be payback from nurse aides, who appear to be shorthanded much of the time but who do most of the work in nursing homes. Working as an aide, Gass (2004: 162–163) explains his infuriation when other employees do not help with something that is officially not their job, stating,

> Another aide and I were left to feed twenty-seven helpless residents in the front dining hall while two office ladies found an empty dining table and proceeded to chat and have lunch. I suggested to them, since they are nice ladies, that they might like to help out in a pinch. I did not know how they could enjoy their visit while seated amid so many stolid people with plates of food gelling before their eyes.

In our observations, similar situations in nursing homes involve staff failing to help with normal bodily functions and personal-hygiene issues. On several occasions, we have seen residents in facilities stranded in wheelchairs wanting someone to roll them to another part of the facility, only to have administrative employees pass them up seemingly oblivious to relocation requests. Stannard (1973) even argues that top-level workers sometimes see resident abuse, but since hands-on care is not technically their job, they look the other way. Backing up this point, we find that cohesion among aides, inadvertently created by staff separation boundaries, sometimes leads to the cover-up of abuse. Similar to accounts of police abuse, allegiance to the fellow workers supersedes whistle blowing. In this case, workers do not hide misconduct behind a badge-oriented blue wall of silence but rather behind a soiled screen of scrubs.

Nursing homes need staff separation at times due to laws ensuring that long-term care workers have the training needed to provide resident care. For example, in the situation described above, the two workers eating their lunch contended that they could not help feed residents because the state had not licensed them to do so. However, we have seen many situations where nursing home workers reproduce hierarchical separation when failing to care for residents they legally could care for. They failed to do so because it was not their "duty." In these situations, without realizing it, employees facilitate the ritualistic establishment of staff boundaries that inadvertently leads to unnecessary neglect.

Rules and Resistance

In our study, we define rules as practices and references to official regulations about the way to do something. This includes the internal rules of a facility. It also includes references to bureaucratic government regulations. In the content analysis portion of this research, 601 references to rules appear, making up 26.4 percent of the bureaucratic references. As Foner (1995: 231) indicates, nursing homes are under a "tyranny" of rules and regulations, while Fontana (1978: 130) argues "rules above compassion" is a dominant theme in nursing homes.

If you spend any amount of time in a nursing home, you will quickly discover that there are rules for everything, and residents feel their omnipresent power. One resident told Howsden (1981: 144), "I feel so strangled here. [There are] so many rules and regulations that don't make any sense." Employees share these feelings. Discussing employee attitudes toward rules, Foner (1994:86) explains,

> Resentments ran especially high because, in an effort to upgrade the facility, the new administrator was tightening enforcement of existing rules and adding new ones. A seemingly endless onslaught of new rules affected even the smallest details of work life. One day aides could wear jewelry to work; the next, after a memo went out, only watches, engagement and wedding rings, and small earrings were allowed.

Rules can be good. Many guidelines implemented in the field of long-term care help reduce problems related to neglect and abuse. Employees tell horror stories of a time when staff could easily take advantage of residents because requirements for everything from food and bathing to staffing did not exist. However, rules become problematic when they become an end in themselves. It is then that employees lose sight of the original goal of the organization. We worry that this is what has happened in nursing homes as the emphasis has shifted away from providing care to making sure employees do not drift from regulatory guidelines.

With nursing homes, the informal goal often seems to be "do things by the book." This creates a strain between the concept of compassion and compliance. Consider bathing: We once came across a resident striving for some autonomy and dignity who wanted to take a bath without help. Because of the resident's limited mobility, laws restricted this practice on the assumption that the resident would always be better off with staff help.

We take the intention well; however, rules like this unintentionally create an RSP that does not favor independence as a form of quality of life for residents. This does not mean that paraplegic residents should always be able to bathe themselves if they want to, but we should recognize that not all nursing home residents are paraplegic. Another remarkable example of rules over compassion involves a situation in our content analysis related to state surveyors.

For a long time, a group of men would congregate every day in the activity room in a specific area where a group of chairs was across from the wide doorway to the dining room at Linda Manor nursing home in Northampton, MA. In a ritualized display of community, they would take turns loudly and humorously announcing the names of dietary aides as they emerged from the kitchen. They had a great time interacting with employees and other residents at this designated spot. The state survey team came in and indicated that the location of the chairs violated rules and put a large dining room table in their place. The men moved their spot to another location at the expense of their physical comfort. Their new area was not located across from the dining room opening, so they had to strain their necks to see which aide was emerging in order to make their announcements (Kidder 1993). Was it more important that a group of institutionalized men were socializing and having a good time, or that a table was where the rules said it had to be? Unfortunately, as one aide explains in relation to ambiguous and unnecessary rules, "Regulations seem to ignore the hard realities of nursing homes and focus instead on matters that make no difference whatever to many residents" (Gass 2004: 61).

Aside from formal rules, informal rules also dictate care in nursing homes. For example, nursing aides have unwritten rules of their own. Unfortunately, we found several situations where aides would comment on informal rules directly related to abuse. In one situation, an aide scalded with hot bath water a senile resident who had cursed at her. The perceived problem was not that the employee had burned a resident, but rather that the resident was incoherent. Implying that the scalding was intentional, another aide said the person should have known that "crazy patients are not punished for cursing aides" (Stannard 1973: 338). It seems that facilities providing care to people would not accept such informal rules, but when informal rules dictate that employees should keep their emotional distance, it is easy to see how abuse is more likely to occur. Lopez (2006a) explains that in a facility he studied, administrators had informal rules that nurses and aides could not talk about their personal lives to residents. Moreover, if a resident did something to upset an employee, it was inappropriate for the worker to talk calmly to the resident about it. This causes two problems. First, it creates a boundary of personalization between residents and staff. Second, it inadvertently creates situations where nurses and aides repress their anger until it is more than they can emotionally handle, which subsequently can lead to physical and verbal explosions.

From a functional perspective, informal rules related to resident punishment and emotional disconnection help to maintain the smooth operation of nursing homes. In turn, nurse aides act as *ritual enforcers* (see Knottnerus, Van Delinder, and Wolynetz, 2010). We believe acceptance of actions such as the aforementioned scalding, along with the misuse of physical restraints and medication and even the ability to regulate television viewing, allow staff an unwarranted level of control in their daily work rituals. The informal demand to keep residents emotionally distant also helps workers objectify them, subsequently easing their ability to carry out abusive sanctions. Under these circumstances, when residents are compliant, we view them as *ritual adjusters* complying with bureaucratic goals and viewed by employees in a positive light. Situations involving residents we call *ritual resisters* are different. Ritual resisters reject the bureaucratic tug toward an emotionless existence and fight for some form of identity.

For instance, they may use personal narratives that involve strategic communication with staff members. They will tell them about their childhood, work experiences, or family relationships to build an emotional bridge (for more, see Paterniti 2000). However, this does not always work. As a last resort, residents may engage in *ritual dissent*. Here, they symbolically protest the enforcement of rules by nursing home workers in a variety of ways. This includes anything from intentionally appearing incontinent to refusing to eat.

Lopez (2006a) discusses a situation where an aide spent more than 15 minutes cleaning and dressing a resident. The resident, who was continent, waited until the aide was finished and then defecated all over herself, so the aide would have to repeat the entire process. Vesperi (1983: 233) contends that this happens all the time to unpopular employees and provides dissatisfied residents with the ability to leave unfavorable caretakers "severely demoralized and convinced that they are engaged in a futile, thankless enterprise."

Documentation and Dehumanization

We define documentation as any aspect of nursing home life expressed in written form. This includes paperwork meeting legal or regulatory requirements. With the content analysis portion of this research, 552 references to rituals involving documentation appear, making up 24.2 percent of the bureaucratic references. This indicates the sources frequently referenced RSPs involving documentation.

In one source, an administrator comments "there is so much of it there is little time left to do anything else" (Farmer 1996: 20). Another worker in the same source explains, "An abundance of tedious paperwork and documentation is the norm and not the exception" (Farmer 1996: 97). In facilities, we observed that documents obviously consume nursing staff. They shape the way staff thinks, speaks, and provides care. Coming off a stint working as a nurse's aide, Diamond (1992: 160) points out:

> Staff continually cursed at being overwhelmed with paperwork. Kenny once waved his hand at the whole row of binders containing these records. "Oh, they're just a formality," he said. They were a formality with force—made of forms and forming the contours of the job, both in doing the prescribed work and in certifying that it had been done ... Sometimes they formed the way we spoke.
>
> A nursing assistant once approached a charge nurse who had been at work at this home for two years. Resident Frances Wasserman, who lost her purse, had now been at the home for two months and was crying out loudly in her room. "Is there anything I can do for her?" asked the nursing assistant ... "Oh," said the nurse, immersed in the medications checklist, "don't worry about it."

Diamond (1992: 131) also tells the story of how one day a nurse pointed over his head to a sign that stated "If It's Not Charted, It Didn't Happen." One of our interviewees, a nursing home director of care who primarily supervises nurses and aides, echoes this issue. Asked if there was a lot of documentation necessary for her position, she stated:

> That's an understatement. [On the other hand], for your average person it may feel like [a lot of paperwork]. But, if you ever have to recall [something you did to a resident] you feel like there was never enough. You gotta write down the pills they take, when they take them. If something was to happen and you had to recall that

information, [it is good to have] somebody's complete life story for the past seven years. I mean, most people have an average of 20 pills a day. You have to give the right pills to the right person. It is a continuous watch for somebody's life.

With these points in mind, it appears documentation provides a medical rationale for dealing with residents, while at the same time helping to turn them into objects of labor. We deal with objectification in detail in the next chapter. Regardless, here it is relevant to point out that when a person views other people as objects, it is easier to victimize them. Consider serial killers. Serial killers are believed to target people they do not know, such as random prostitutes, because it makes it easier to assault and torture them. When serial killers see victims as nonhuman, it prevents them from viewing the person harmed as a mother, father, or someone's child, and their horrendous acts do not have as much of an impact on their conscience (Egger and Egger 2003).

So, what kind of documentation leads to dehumanization? Consider the ritual use of B.M. books that keep track of resident bowel movements (Kidder 1993). They turn what many would consider a personal act into a quantitative measurement. Legally and medically, it may be necessary to keep up with the condition of residents with documentation procedures; however, we have to consider the drawback of writing everything down when it turns residents into meager work objects, especially if it is possible that it is a process contributing to abuse and neglect.

The Effectiveness of Efficiency

We define efficiency as demands to behave quickly and effectively. It is an essential goal of all complex organization management. This is particularly true of Medicaid-dependent facilities with little budget slack. Therefore, it is not surprising that in our content analysis, rituals related to efficiency appeared 265 times, making up 11.6 percent of the bureaucratic items in the data.

Consistent with most low-wage, service-based employment, our observations confirm the idea that nursing home workers, specifically nurses and aides, have a thumb of efficiency constantly pressing down on them. We have visited residents in their rooms and on many occasions witnessed aides rush in, distribute medications, fill water cups, and zoom out of the door without saying much at all, if even anything, to the other people there. Based on the pressure of organizational dynamics, you really cannot blame them. As one aide states, "Every morning is a head-on collision against time. I am learning to be efficient and gentle in a hurry" (Gass 2004: 13). The main reason for the desire for greater efficiency is understaffing. As Fontana (1978: 130) concludes based on his observations in a nursing home:

> There were usually a minimal number of aides on the ward, and in order to meet administrative demands the aides would accomplish their daily assignments as quickly as possible. The patient was scrubbed, washed, turned over, rinsed—and the aides were ready for the next patient. Feeding the patients followed the same course. In the rushed meal hour, food was shoved down open mouths or splattered on closed mouths as the aides carried on without missing a beat … it mattered little to them since the goal of efficiency was seemingly more important.

The director of care interviewed, who was in fact once an aide, believes that efficiency demands coupled with low staff numbers is the root of quality care problems. She indicated to us that cost saving trumps good care saying, "The state requires minimum staffing, and if they require five [aides on one floor], but you could [do a better job] with ten, most places would have just five."

Residents are well aware of this phenomenon. We have heard residents comment on not knowing the names of the caretakers, or just not knowing much about them. Bernice Lewis, a resident at a facility in Kansas, wrote in her diary:

> I wish the girls [aides] were not so rushed. I know they have a lot to do but they bustle in here in the mornings and you can feel their impatience. I always try to be ready for them and think of what I need while they are here. But we older people are slow and sometimes it's hard to get moving. It makes us nervous when they are always racing around. (Hale 2005: 169)

Even if aides want to resist the temptation to rush through their tasks, organizational rules can impede their desires. As alluded to earlier, nursing home rules sometimes prohibit them from building personal relationships. Lopez (2006a: 144–145), explains how livid a supervisor was upon finding aides having personal conversations with residents:

> The aides, seeing Cindy, jumped up immediately, caught in the act of socializing with residents instead of working on them. It was clear they knew they'd been caught doing something wrong. She gave them a written disciplinary warning that would go in their personal files ... for being caught sitting. Afterward she groused to me, "I understand this job isn't always fun, but when you are here you're being paid to work, not to sit around and gossip."

One thing our research is clear on: Most of the time a good worker in a nursing home is not a worker that affectionately cares for residents, but one who quickly executes required tasks. Foner (1994: 60) explains:

> Ms. James was typically the first nursing aide in the dayroom at lunchtime getting residents ready to eat. She was a fast worker.

She finished her "bed and body" work early and was punctilious about getting her paperwork done neatly and on time. Ms. James's attitude toward dressing, bathing, and feeding patients was much the same as her attitude toward her other chores. She was determined to get them all done quickly, whether patients liked it or not. Residents in her view had no choice but to take prescribed medicines, eat so they would not lose weight or be forced to go on tube feeding, or "do a BM" so they would not get impacted. She had no tolerance for patients' resistance, which slowed her down. In fact, Ms. James was proud that she could get patients to eat and "do a BM" so they would not get impacted. I overheard her explain, indeed justify, her approach to one of the therapists: "Schmidt eats for me, but if anyone hears me they're gonna get me for patient abuse."

As with the rules category, here it does not matter how you do something, just that you do it quickly. In the previous example, this applies to feeding, but we also want to note that it applies to other processes as well, such as dressing residents. Certain sources indicate that sometimes staff put on resident gowns backwards, and not because they make mistakes in the clothing process, but rather they put gowns on backwards so they can more quickly clean residents when they soil themselves (see Kayser-Jones 1981). This may intentionally speed up the workday, but we think it also serves to dehumanize people who expect to be dressed in a proper manner. Efficiency might be effective if you are producing something in a factory, but is it counter-productive when you are trying to provide a holistic health care experience? As a *GQ* writer points out in a recent issue, "More than a generation into our national obsession with efficiency, people are realizing that the notion of squeezing more productivity out of fewer resources is the economic equivalent of the perpetual motion machine ... and I hate that efficiency has displaced quality as the ultimate American ideal" (Donahue 2008: 290).

Meetings for the Sake of Meetings

Most Americans politically participate in, are educated by, or work for a bureaucratic organization. Therefore, many of us are familiar with the phenomenon of meetings. The content analysis portion of this research was open to emerging themes, so we developed an "other" category for miscellaneous themes that emerged during our coding of literature. In regard to rituals of bureaucracy in nursing homes, the most prominent theme involved meetings.

It would be hard to find someone who has not sat in a meeting and wondered why the meeting was necessary in the first place. We believe just having meetings for the sake of having meetings serves to legitimize the existence of bureaucracy. Why do people in bureaucracies meet so much? In part, because that is what you do when you belong to a bureaucracy. The senior author for this book has attended academic meetings for more than ten years and keeps a notebook of important meeting points directly related to his job requirements. Not knowing if it is funny or sad, he will often show it to new faculty members who are nervous about attending one of their first formal congregations with colleagues. So, what is funny, or maybe sad? The notebook has just a few lines written on the first page and a clown doodled on one page halfway through. This begs the question: Could people in bureaucracies be doing something more productive if they had fewer meetings? Nursing home employees certainly think so.

Coupling the previously mentioned issue of documentation with the theme of meetings, one activity director explains, "All nursing home staff have so much paperwork to do, they spend about 50 percent of their time charting and 10 to 20 percent attending mandatory meetings. So, this only leaves about 30 to 40 percent of their time to spend with residents" (Poxon 2004: 81). An aide elaborates, stating, "When you have too many meetings in a day, they take you from your direct work and take your time away from the patient and slow you up" (Foner 1994: 73). Therefore, evidence indicates that the result of meetings designed to increase quality care for residents ironically can have the opposite effect. When a day has too many meetings, employees who provide direct care for residents must rush back to their areas and hurry to complete tasks and paperwork. Once again, we get the message that bureaucracy is more important than resident care.

We feel it is important to note that meetings not only serve to legitimize bureaucratic existence, but also reinforce power boundaries in nursing homes. In this area, meetings involving employees and the families of residents are relevant. In one situation in our data, a pastor tells the story of how he felt his wife was not receiving the appropriate level of care, so he decided to bring her a mild pain reliever from home. The staff, who he claims always wanted to hold his wife's personal care meetings spontaneously when he was visiting her just to keep the control in their hands, pulled him into an administrative office one day. Several employees were there facing off against only him. They accused him of trying to give his own medications to his wife in order to kill her. They also notified him that they contacted the local prosecuting attorney and that he was not to remove his wife from the facility (for more see Mollette 2001). Legal compromise led to a peaceful resolution of the accusation, which had little substantive evidence backing it up. However, people should be aware that nursing homes sometimes use meetings to enhance control over residents and their family members.

Organizational Variation

Our content analysis data reveals a certain degree of organizational variation because we find a higher frequency of staff separation and rule-based rituals in nonprofit sources. On the other hand, the frequency of references to documentation and efficiency rituals in for-profit and nonprofit sources is very similar. In terms of salience, examples that emphasized the importance of staff separation, rules, documentation, and efficiency exist in both for-profit and nonprofit sources. This leads us to conclude that nursing homes, regardless of ownership type, struggle to survive under the looming shadow of bureaucratic dynamics. Moreover, both types are in a battle between bureaucratic and quality of care goals. As this chapter illustrates, unfortunately the former can win out, leaving residents to suffer.

In the movie *Wedding Crashers,* the two lead characters ditch their calculated rules for behavior and find that the dehumanization of people can have serious consequences. It not only leads to poor treatment of others, but it leaves the person who manages relationships guided by rules above compassion with a deflated level of self-worth (Faber and Fisher 2005). In a world saturated with bureaucracy, we think that lesson is an important one.

CHAPTER 5
PRODUCTS NOT PEOPLE

The whole drive of western culture, the part of it
which is serious, is towards an extreme objectification. It's carried to the point where the human
subject is treated almost as if it's dirt in the works
of a watch.

Henry Flynt

Henry Flynt, musician-turned-philosopher, used the preceding
quote in reference to his feelings of the art world (Home 1989).
His words are quite applicable to the elder care catastrophe. They
echo Max Weber's concern that bureaucracy, as a key component
of western culture, takes the emotional attachments out of interaction and simply turns people into mechanical cogs in a large,
lifeless machine.

In this chapter, we analyze the link between bureaucracy and
the emotional neglect of nursing home residents. On the premise
that employees ritualistically view residents as unemotional work
products and not people, it explains some basic types of emotional
neglect we believe are prevalent in nursing homes.

Emotional Neglect in Nursing Home Care

As Table 5.1 illustrates, 346 ritualized acts of emotional neglect appear in the content analysis portion of our research. They include objectification, inadequate compassion, and spiritual neglect.

The Saturation of Objectification

The previous chapter briefly alluded to objectification, but here it is a category of emotional neglect deserving attention all on its own. For classification purposes, we define objectification as any situation where nursing home employees treat residents as impersonal, material items. This involves, for example, nursing home employees ritualistically referring to residents by room number or ailment instead of by their names. With our content analysis, 182 references to objectification appear, making up 52.6 percent of ritualized practices in this category.

Sociologists discuss the process of objectification in a variety of ways. Objectification often results from people in power having the ability to label and control others. Consider the objectification that takes place when someone enters prison, a total institution that much of the nursing home literature ironically refers to when describing resident experiences. People provided power by

Table 5.1 Frequencies for Emotional Neglect Rituals

Subdivision	Number	Percent
Objectification	182	52.6
Compassion transgressions	116	33.5
Spiritual negligence	48	13.9
Total	346	100.0

organizational employment strip you down, search your orifices for hidden objects, tell you what to wear and how to wear it, tell you what you can eat, when to wake up, when to sleep, and what your identification number will be. You are no longer a name, but an object lost in a maze of rules and regulations with little command over your life. Those controlling your everyday actions will have little concern about who, or what, you used to be (Ross and Richards 2002). You are no longer just "Bob" or "Mary," but to those in power, "inmate."

That sounds a lot like what happens when you enter a nursing home. Joan Retsinas's mother lived in a nursing home for an extended period. From a sociological perspective, she explains how objectification plays out by way of nurse aides. Retsinas (1986: 90) states:

> Whatever the route, however, the individual becomes a "resident" … that identity overshadows, even eclipses, any prior identity. In nursing homes, people are identified by disability, by nursing needs, by room number, perhaps even by physician. Mrs. Smith becomes "the self-care patient on Unit 3," or "the woman with MS," or "one of Dr. Jones's patients." Mr. Morgan becomes the "terminal case in Room 26."

Facilities do attempt to hold on to some aspects of residents' personal identity. It is not as if all nursing homes have room numbers with signs below that simply say "cancer" or "bed sores." Many put the name of residents on the door for identification purposes along with a photograph of the person. However, it is often just the last name, and the photographs we have seen tend to be ones from the person's earlier years. We think that is a good practice, because it can fight off objectification by letting employees see the person when their skin was tighter and their body was functioning better. However, it can also serve as a reminder of what may never return. We should note that nursing home aides sometimes indicate that keeping a level of emotional distance from residents is a defense mechanism. They do not want to get close to residents they know will eventually leave or pass away; however, some facilities have explicit policies in place that require aides to keep their emotional distance from residents (Lopez 2006a).

Because aides spend the most time with nursing home residents, it is easy to point the finger at aides as the only people objectifying residents. However, we find that objectification in the nursing homes has few boundaries. We find administrative employees have their hands in the objectification jar as well. Diamond (1992: 176) describes his realization of this issue when he was working as an aide and conversing with an administrator:

> "How are things going for you up here?" "Oh, not bad," I responded with a slight chuckle, nodding toward [a resident]. "I kinda like a lot of the people." As the elevator doors opened and she backed in, she nodded in apparent agreement with me. "Yes," ... "they're a good team. Very professional." The head nurse's assumption that by "people" I meant staff served as an example of a certain attitude that dominated the settings. [Residents] living there were the receivers of service, more acted upon than actors, whose ability to act was reduced not only by their own incapacities but by administrative definitions.

Administrators are aware of the power their definitions have. The senior author was visiting a facility near his home one balmy March afternoon where an activity director agreed to an interview. She was discussing, in a way implying she viewed residents more as a commodity than living beings, how the facility's biggest concern was filling more beds. The conversation finally turned to the quality of life for people in the facility. Reflecting the objectifying tone of medical lingo, she continually called people in the facility "patients," would catch herself, and then call them "residents at the home." The objectification of residents also ties into resident stratification. We do not believe this is always a bad idea. Activity directors imply their job is more effective when low-functioning residents and high-functioning ones have different recreational outlets. It is also safer for staff to separate certain residents from others. For example, it is a common practice in nursing homes to have "wings" dedicated to people with severe cognitive impairments. Many facilities have "Alzheimer's Units" designed to isolate people with mental deficiencies. When spending time in facilities that do not stratify on the basis of mental health issues, we hear stories about residents with cognitive impairments stealing, physically abusing, or even sexually assaulting others. One resident the senior author visited on several occasions in a facility located in rural Oklahoma provides some insight.

Chloe was born and raised in Abilene, TX. She experienced major health problems, including two strokes, after her husband James died. She moved to Oklahoma to stay in a nursing home close to her daughter. When she was not talking about her childhood experiences picking cotton or how much she missed James, she was on the lookout for fellow residents with the potential to victimize her. She was particularly concerned with fellow residents who had severe dementia. Her nursing home did not separate them from other residents. At the displeasure of employees, she kept a chain running across the doorway to her room. Chloe once stated:

> This chain isn't meant to keep me in, but to keep "them" out. They used to be called "crazy people." Now the doctors have given them a new name [Alzheimer's]. Some people lose their mind in here, but I've kept mine. Jason, I'm just walking in the land of crazy people.

She implied that residents had been in her room while she was asleep and taken some of her things. After visiting with her a few times and hearing her talk about her own struggles with memory, it seemed like the chain served more of a symbolic function. Chloe wanted a barrier, not only for protection, but also so that she could see something that physically separated her from what she did not want to be. Therefore, it seems the separation of residents based on functioning has multiple positive purposes for residents and employees alike. However, we think this stratification can go too far. Consider the practice of color-coding.

With color-coding, employees put colored dots on the outside of resident doors to act as visual keys allowing them to recall a resident's health status. Should nursing homes allow employees to orient their awareness of a resident's condition by glancing at a colored sticker? Moreover, should people who do not work for the facility, or even other residents who are knowledgeable of the color-coding system, be able to identify someone's health problems by glancing at a door? Since the passage of the Health Insurance Portability and Accountability Act (HIPAA) in 1996, and specifically privacy rules that addressed disclosure issues in the health field that took effect in 2003, we have not seen or heard much about color-coding. However, in our discussions with nursing home employees, stories about similar practices do come up.

Another issue relating to objectification involves facility closures. Of course, it is important for state survey teams to come into a facility and analyze its operation, but many people fail to realize what happens if the state shuts down a nursing home. In many instances, states will give facilities a short time to transfer residents. Like cattle shipped off to different feed lots, residents are loaded into ambulances and sent to other nursing homes with extra room. Of course, with the other homes there is a premium on gaining Medicare residents because they ensure a steady flow of income (Poxon 2004).

The saturation of objectification is not something isolated in nursing homes. We think aspects of ageism contribute to the objectification of the elderly even when not institutionalized. As Gass (2004: 83) explains, "Time so transforms a body that we often forget that there is still a real person hiding behind all those wrinkles and thick glasses." Regardless, we think bureaucratic forces cannot help but multiply this phenomenon, especially when facilities encourage employees to limit their emotional connections with residents. It just undermines humanity.

Lack of Compassion

We identify compassion transgressions as ritualized actions involving staff failing to exhibit emotional awareness of and desire to relieve resident suffering. This includes employees who do not help residents with personal items, although they acknowledge their requests; do not provide food when residents are hungry; and discuss residents' physical conditions without any semblance of compassion. With our content analysis, we found 116 references to compassion transgressions, making up 33.5 percent of the emotional neglect analyzed. Kayser-Jones (1981: 49) provides an interesting example:

> Ninety-nine-year-old Mr. White, a bachelor, is alone in the world. His only visitor is a woman who has been appointed by the court to be his guardian. "Pull up a chair and sit down," he immediately suggested as I entered the room. As I started to offer him a glass of water, I found the pitcher empty. I filled it with ice water and gave him some. "Thank you, that was wonderful," he said. "One boy used to come and give me water, but nobody comes any more. They are all so cruel to me. I asked a nurse for a towel to clean my glasses and

she handed me a wet one. I said, this towel is wet and she said it's good enough for you. Some of the boys who mop the floor are nice to me, but the nurses don't talk to me. They walk by the door, but nobody stops to talk with me."

To many people, getting a fresh cup of water is a taken-for-granted task. For the institutionalized, it can be a treat that creates an emotional spark. One nursing home resident the senior author visited with several times for this research had a roommate that loved it when aides would bring her fresh water. She once commented that her roommate was having problems getting fresh water, though the aides knew it lifted her spirits. She felt like an aide mocked her roommate's request for water one day. She stated, "[The aide] came in here and brought her some water in a pitcher with an empty cup ... [They know] she can't even lift her arms, let alone a pitcher of water!"

It is sometimes hard to decipher when employees know what a resident can and cannot do. Regardless, it seems clear that whether they are intentional or not, compassion transgressions take an emotional toll. Sue Hale's mother Bernice was in a facility near Wichita, Kansas. Hale was visiting her mother one day and witnessed a compassion transgression first hand. She (2005: 172) notes:

> The [aide] came into the room one day, and it would be a day when mom's spirits were sagging, and she started questioning why Mother couldn't stand at least on one leg when being moved from the bed to the wheelchair. That way it would only take one aide to get her out of bed. With only one leg in a brace, it did look as if the other leg was strong enough to bear mom's weight. "I explained to her I had a stress fracture in my left leg and I wasn't supposed to stand on it but she kept saying it would be easier on them if I did," Mom said. Mother was torn between being tempted to try to stand on her "good" leg and being afraid of risking it for fear she would fall ...

She said she must have looked depressed [about it] at dinner that evening in the dining room because one of the nurses came over and asked her what was wrong.

With compassion transgression rituals, staff will even comment on how they want problematic residents to die. Vesperi (1983: 236) gives an account where workers discussed the possibility of a resident's suffocation and one commented, "What difference does it make? That's much less for us to do." Relating back to bureaucratic issues discussed in Chapter 4, we also find paperwork can whittle a resident's well-being down to a few descriptive words that, if taken at face value, cancel out the possibility of the person even experiencing emotions. As an aide, Gass (2004) wanted to know more about a resident for whom he was caring. He consulted the five-foot-tall, 60-pound elderly woman's chart for some details, since he knew she spent most of the day in her bed suffering from anxiety. When he read her chart, staff only had one word written: "unremarkable."

Mismanaging Beliefs and Morals

We define spiritual negligence as the failure to acknowledge and maintain a resident's sacred beliefs or moral feelings. We do not think spirituality is limited to the participation in, and practice of, religion. For us it concerns any intangible aspect of emotional well-being, including factors associated with personal loss and death. This includes failing to acknowledge resident grief after a death or handling a resident death in an unconcerned manner. With the content analysis part of our research, this category appears 48 times, making up 13.9 percent of the emotional neglect rituals examined.

At first glance, some of the sources used in our content analysis, especially the nonprofit, religious ones, give an impression of higher levels of spiritual support. Residents speak about the importance of religion and access to worship services. With respect to a Catholic-based facility, one resident stated, "The ability to have that chapel and to go to Mass after you have worked in the world for 70 years like I did, or 50 years ... you appreciate that chapel" (O'Brien 1989: 47). Regardless, we found as many references to spiritual negligence in nonprofit sources as in secular, for-profit ones. Howsden's (1981: 61) research provides us with an example:

> Is that minister still preaching? It's sure getting close to medication time and people should be getting back to their rooms. [The aide replied] this happened last week, too. They are such a long-winded bunch ... maybe someone should mention to them that their service lasts too long. [The nurse said] these people don't need that much religion.

Here, we see another link between bureaucracy and emotional neglect. Nurses and aides may have disdain for religious practices because they throw a kink into the work routine. Downplaying the importance of religion chips away at the spiritual side of residents' lives. Nonetheless, it is important to keep in mind that residents can display actions of spiritual neglect against employees as well. Gass (2004: 103) overheard a resident and nurse discussing another resident's death when the nurse said, "We shouldn't be sad cause the Bible says we should rejoice when a soul goes to our true home in heaven," and the resident replied, "Ah, don't bother me with the Bible. The Bible is full of shit."

In regard to death issues, we also find interesting themes. Outside of nursing home walls, sociologists note that circles of death notification exist. With the typical scenario, death news follows a specific path. Hospital personnel are the first to know, then the coroner, immediate family, other relatives, and then friends.

Finally, acquaintances and community members hear about the death (DeSpelder and Strickland 2009). This common trajectory is, however, changing. Whereas telephone calls and newspaper obituaries used to be the dominant media for death news, the Internet is the new outlet. The Internet was the first medium to report the recent death of pop icon Michael Jackson, but it is not just instrumental in the delivery of death news on the famous. The senior author recently taught a class on death and dying and was astonished to find out how many of the students had learned of the death of friends and family through MySpace or Facebook pages. No doubt, the wave of the future will probably involve sending tweets to others up until your last breath. Regardless, we know that death news works differently behind nursing home walls. This is, perhaps, due to two factors: bureaucratic divisions and a lack of desire to acknowledge death.

As for bureaucratic divisions, multiple pockets of people hinder the information flow. For example, the senior author went to a facility to visit a resident he befriended only to find her room empty. He asked a resident walking by what happened to her. The resident said, "She's dead." Attempting to confirm this, he turned to staff. He asked an aide. She said, "I think she went to the hospital for a few days." Not believing her statement, which came across with a tone of uncertainty, he asked the director of nursing on duty. She implied nothing was wrong with her and she was in her room as usual. The aide ended up being the one with accurate information.

With the lack of desire to acknowledge death, employees, perhaps due to the normalization of dealing with mortality issues, fail to recognize someone passing or its effects on others. This could have positive benefits. In terms of emotional well-being, you do not want a large number of elderly people housed together to be bombarded with death scenes and information. On the other hand, it seems odd to just ignore death issues or treat them in a callous way. Shield (1988: 70) describes this scenario that occurred at a Jewish facility where she spent a considerable amount of time:

> When the death finally occurs, the room is closed, the physician is called so the body may be "pronounced," the next of kin is notified, the personal effects are picked up, and the body is taken to the funeral home. Staff time is occupied with sanitation and paperwork following the death. Meanwhile, the news of the death travels quickly and stealthily among residents, though there is little or no staff disclosure to them. There was no memorial service, there was no notice on the bulletin boards in the hallways; there was no place to mention the event in the resident newsletter, and there was no kaddish (the Jewish prayer for the dead).

When someone dies, employees sometimes act as if the person never lived. Savishinsky (1991: 210) says, "You see them one week and then, within a few days, someone new has moved into their room. It's almost like they did not exist." This leaves surviving residents without emotional closure and fosters a coldhearted approach to their condition. Discussing a situation where a resident passed away, Kidder (1993: 212) notes:

> Earl died in his room the following morning. Across from the nurses' station sat the usual lineup of residents in wheelchairs. Earl's roommate sat across the way, in his wheelchair in front of the nurse's station. "At least he didn't suffer," said Earl's roommate through his sobs. Behind the counter a nurse stood holding the telephone, saying to someone in the kitchen, "I want to tell you that Earl Duncan just died. Just so you won't send us a tray for him."

Kidder (1993) goes on to explain that in order to notify residents, the facility did announce deaths with a marker board located in the nursing home kitchen. It would have the resident's name printed with a marker followed by the word "deceased." There was also an obituary board in the main hall. It listed the person's name and just a line or two worth of description. Typically, these obituaries referred only to the dead person's appreciation for a good bingo game.

When it comes to death in nursing homes, it is just bureaucratic-based, business as usual. Glenn Mollette (2001: 86) was taken aback when his wife, whose room at the nursing home had a view of the front door, told him almost every day, "They took another dead body out of here today. They pulled right up to the front of the building and I watched two men load another dead body. Is that what I have to look forward to?" This way of handling death can be a bit of a shock to family members when dealing with nursing home employees. Hale (2005) was walking around a nursing home in which she was considering placing her mother when the administrator quickly threw two odd questions at her. One was whether she had a problem with employees using physical restraints to tie her mother down. The other was what funeral home she preferred. She said she almost left when she heard the second question since she did not plan on her mom dying anytime soon. Is that just being practical or brutish?

Not a Laughing Matter

The content analysis theme that emerged during our coding of initial categories centers on ridicule rituals. These rituals include situations where staff openly make fun of residents and their conditions. Again, we did not systematically look for these rituals from the beginning of our content analysis. We noticed these rituals well after our coding of the three main forms of emotional neglect just discussed was taking place. Nonetheless, we believe they are worth mentioning and certainly deserve attention in future research.

Some of the examples of ritual ridicule include situations involving general matters where employees engage in laughter about things that not everyone would interpret as laughing matters. For example, Gass (2004: 127) details an instance involving a resident taking a shower:

> On my very first day of work here I helped to give Walter a shower. The maneuver required three people—one to wash him and two to restrain him by gripping a towel twisted around both wrists. At the time he looked like a rabid raccoon. Deep-purple bruises from a bad fall and two black eyes had transformed his face into a primitive war mask. He was cursing and fighting with all his might. Aides were laughing and dodging. . . .

Vesperi (2003: 98–99) reveals her cousin's attitude toward staff name-calling in a conversation pertaining to his opinion of aides:

> "They can't stand to look at me. I'm ridiculed as 'Santa Claus' or 'Adams.' They made a picture of some guy by the name of Adams. He was supposed to be a, a man of the country, a hill man. 'Fuzzy.' They call me 'Fuzzy.'" T.D. was clearly unfamiliar with the television program *Grizzly Adams*. I was unsure whether knowledge of its content would have assuaged or increased his outrage at the comparison. "That's not good, to ridicule anybody," T.D. continued. "That breaks your spirit."

Regardless of general laughter and name-calling, we did see two prominent areas of ritual ridicule. They focus on incontinence and sexuality. Kayser-Jones (1981: 47) discusses how one nurse found humor in a volunteer's reaction to a resident's inability to control urination:

> Mr. Thomas always sat in a particular location in the hallway. One evening I saw him struggling to get out of his wheelchair. Sensing he needed a urinal, I called the nurse. "Oh, that's all right," she

assured me. "Don't worry about him; he has two spots right here in the hallway where he urinates every day." The expression on my face was one of shock and disbelief as I watched the man publicly urinate on the carpet in the hallway. "What's the matter," laughed the nurse, "is it too much for you?"

Public urination is a major violation of cultural norms. One thing that classifies us as adult, if not human, is the ability to control and contain our bodily fluids (Mitteness and Barker 1995). When nursing home employees make fun of incontinence, it degrades and further dehumanizes residents suffering from incontinence. We believe that making fun of the inability to control and contain bodily fluids helps employees distance themselves from those for whom they provide care. Therefore, ritual ridicule smoothes the emotional distancing process in bureaucratic settings like nursing homes. We believe situations involving the denial of sexuality do the same.

Fontana (1978: 128) describes a sexual humiliation ritual he observed in one nursing home noting that "big John" walked around with his pants undone pleasuring himself while "aides [just] laughed at him." He further noted that big John once had another resident perform fellatio on him. When staff caught them, they laughed and never even asked the other resident whether she was a willing participant. Why would employees of any organization see this as acceptable? We believe it is because employees who view residents as objects do not see them as having the ability to be sexual. Therefore, they sometimes treat sexual behavior, such as masturbation or sexual contact, as amusing instead of a basic part of human behavior.

Another bureaucratic requirement backing up beliefs of asexuality among residents involves room separation. Some facilities require married couples to live in separate rooms. Moreover, few facilities provide private areas for intimate contact for sexually active residents and loved ones who come to visit. This is unfortunate, because studies show older people who maintain intimate relations report higher levels of well-being (McKenzie 2000).

Organizational Variation

Concerning rituals of emotional neglect in our content analysis data, we found high frequencies of objectification and compassion transgressions. The accounts we examined do not create the impression that nursing home employees intentionally place a great emphasis on promoting emotional neglect. However, we can note that a majority of examples comprising these categories did come from for-profit sources. Though we found fewer examples of spiritual negligence compared to the other categories, we do feel that the examples analyzed imply that employees in both for-profit and nonprofit homes place a great value on being able to suppress residents' feelings toward religion, and more particularly death. This is not a great surprise because nursing homes operate on more of a medical basis, which seems to stand at odds with ideas, such as faith, that relate to supernatural beliefs.

Based on our findings, we have little doubt that emotional neglect is a big part of the elder care catastrophe. We believe that in nursing homes, employees are objectifying residents, not providing them with adequate levels of compassion, not respecting their spiritual well-being, and sometimes ridiculing them for physical conditions out of their control. Some employees in nursing homes provide care to the elderly while viewing them as emotionless, inanimate objects akin to Henry Flynt's dirt at the bottom of a watch. Unfortunately, the elderly have to sit in their own private hells just passing time watching dirt collect and blow away with few people acknowledging it existed in the first place.

CHAPTER 6
TRANQUILIZING THE TROUBLEMAKERS

Zoologists and social scientists may ultimately
find a blending of their professional areas of
studies.

James H. Boren

In 2007 on Christmas Day in some San Francisco mall, Santa
Claus was handing out presents to children. At the same time, a
243-pound escaped Siberian tiger was using his claws to maul a
17-year-old San Jose boy at the San Francisco Zoo. Police killed
the tiger soon after arriving at the scene, but the boy was already
dead (Piller and Reiterman 2007). Visitor deaths are not common with zoo escapes. Usually, the main escapees are of the tame
variety, mostly birds. However, dangerous animals do experience
brief stints of freedom. In June 2009, a gorilla weighing close to
400 pounds climbed out of his enclosure at the Columbia, SC,
Riverbanks Zoo. Employees rushed to the scene ready to tranquil-
ize the troublemaker, but the gorilla hopped back in his exhibit
(Holleman 2009).

Zoos and nursing homes have a few similarities. They have
staff assigned to feed, bathe, and provide other types of general

care. They both contain creatures from the outside world, usually against their own wills. They certainly both have visitors, though we have never heard of a resident mauling a nursing home visitor to death. Finally, they both have escapes. In fact, many nursing homes will put electronic devices on residents they fear will flee. Usually these are for demented residents with the potential to wander out and into danger. While the senior author was working at a nursing home in northeast Arkansas, the facility was buzzing for weeks about a local facility under state investigation where a cognitively-impaired resident wandered away one night and was found the next morning dead in a ditch.

In this chapter, we analyze the link between bureaucracy and the physical maltreatment of nursing home residents. With the idea that nursing homes sometimes promote bureaucratic goals over physical well-being, it focuses on issues relating to medical, personal, and environmental negligence, along with rituals related to bodily harm. We expect nursing home employees to take quality physical care of residents just as zookeepers do for their charges; however, that does not always happen. By the end of this chapter, you will see another common theme between zoos and nursing homes: They both have employees ready to contain unruly creatures that cause disruptions to the everyday work routines, even if physical welfare suffers. Regrettably, gorillas are not the only troublemakers people are tranquilizing.

Physical Maltreatment in Nursing Home Care

As Table 6.1 illustrates, 502 ritualized acts of physical maltreatment appear in the content analysis portion of our research. They include aspects of medical dereliction, personal and environmental negligence, and bodily harm.

Table 6.1 Frequencies for Physical Maltreatment Rituals

Subdivision	Number	Percent
Medical dereliction	144	28.7
Personal negligence	134	26.7
Environmental negligence	117	23.3
Bodily harm	107	21.3
Total	502	100.0

Subpar Service and the Seduction of Sedation

We define rituals of medical dereliction as the failure to deliver medicine and services that have the capacity to help or heal resident's ailments. This includes doctors failing to provide care and nursing staff using pharmaceutical drugs, such as Thorazine, for the sole purpose of controlling a resident's behavior. In these situations, residents do not require medication, but staff will still use it to keep annoying patients from disrupting work. With our content analysis, 144 references to rituals of medical dereliction appear, making up 28.7 percent of the physical maltreatment instances analyzed.

Physicians sometimes refuse to provide medical care for residents believing that doing so is pointless because of their age. Kayser-Jones (1981: 76) recalls, "The nurse in charge of Unit B said that on some occasions when she had suggested glasses or a hearing aid for a patient, the doctor had rejected this suggestion with, 'Oh well, she's old anyhow.'" There are also situations where doctors request specific forms of care and nursing home employees simply do not abide. It may be because they are uncomfortable with a resident's condition. A former aide we collected interview data from told us that she worked in a facility that had a resident with AIDS. Some of the workers did not like to provide the resident care or even feed him. Aides that were more compassionate picked up the unwilling aides' slack and even snuck in burgers for the gentleman from time to time to lift his spirits. However, sometimes the failure of staff to provide doctor-recommended care is more perplexing. Either they simply do not want to do what physicians order or they unintentionally fail to because of other pending duties. Consider Billy Hill's situation.

The senior author collected data from Billy in July of 2009. Not being able to provide his mother with the care she needed in his home after she broke her hip, he put her in a nursing home. She was 83. He hoped she would receive some rehabilitation and her condition would improve. However, after being in the facility for just a few weeks, her hip broke again. Billy says he still is not sure how she broke the hip again. Staff told him she must have done it when she was by herself and that she probably just fell out of her wheelchair. A gerontological psychiatrist told Bill that the second break was too much for her mentally, and her cognitive abilities soon diminished. With respect to her medical care, a couple of instances trouble Billy. He explains:

> There was a specific instance in which an eye doctor had ordered that Mom receive a specific medication for an eye infection four times a day. One day, she did not receive the medication during the day at all, and did not receive it until the evening, when the on-duty nurse only applied it once. Later, I talked to a different nurse about this instance, and it was written up, with the negligent nurse receiving a reprimand. Also ... though previously Mom had twice had to go to the hospital for dehydration, it was rare that water was set by Mom's bedside. I reported this to the isolation wing nurse, but the problem continued. Consequently, I reported this lack of bedside water to the nursing home's chief administrator; he apologized and told me he would handle the situation.

Based on our analysis, we believe the lack of medical attention in some facilities revolves around money. Diamond reports that when working in a nursing home he would tell residents "it costs a lot to take care of sick people these days" (1992: 151). However, he did not believe the administrator in his facility was always appropriately spending on the medical needs of residents. When this happens, it puts employees, specifically aides, in a pinch. It is more common than most people would think for aides to bring medical supplies from home to use on residents. A better aide complained to Diamond (1992: 151) one day stating, "Damn ... I forgot to bring those Epsom salts. Now Violet is not going to be able to soak her foot." Family members also sneak their own medications in from time to time. The facility might be short on medical supplies or not administering them to your liking, but we caution against this practice. Mollette (2001) tried to bring his wife Advil from home and employees accused him of trying to kill his wife with drugs they did not know she was taking. Do not get yourself caught up in a web of legality if you can help it.

Regardless of subpar levels of medical care, sometimes employees provide an overabundance of it. As mentioned, nursing home workers overmedicate residents that cause disruptions to the bureaucratic flow of the workday. Workers label residents "disrupting deviants" even when medications to control them cause the initial problem. Fontana (1978: 128) explains:

> The center exhibited many forms of deviance, which were perpetrated by individual members of the organization but were really done for and normalized in the name of the organization. The goal of the center, a typical one in this respect, was to provide a smooth-running schedule and flow of work, minimizing disturbances and avoiding trouble. What constituted disturbances and trouble was defined by the staff. Hence many deviant acts perpetrated by patients on other patients or by staff members were handled to minimize their hindrance to the running of the organization. Often these acts were normalized in order to avoid stopping the center's smoothly flowing machine.

Therefore if Maria, a wiry old patient, fell heavily to the ground after having been pumped full of Thorazine, the incident was dismissed as the result of an obfuscated mind and deteriorated body.

Other examples of this practice exist in our content analysis sources. They indicate that nurses may officially have control of medication rituals, but aides are really in charge. Sometimes aides even blackmail nurses by refusing to provide care on their wings until the drugging of annoyingly disruptive residents takes place. Nurses in a crunch, with aide shortages and their own bureaucratic constraints, do not have a problem complying. In his classic study on nursing home life, Gubrium (1975: 148) describes the feelings of one nurse after being pressured to administer medications to subdue residents, "As one floor nurse stated to several aides just before leaving for her break, 'Well, I guess I can take my break now. Everyone's sedated.'" Gubrium (1975: 148–149) elaborates:

> Residents do not necessarily enter the Manor with physician's orders for tranquilizers. However, when aides define them as "troublemakers," they get tranquilizers shortly after. Tranquilizers are mostly prescribed "PRN," which means that they may be administered as needed at the discretion of the floor nurses. In practice, however, the discretion involved is that of the aide, who asks for, or reminds a floor nurse of "her need" for a sedative. From start to finish, the prescription and administration of tranquilizers is controlled indirectly by aides.

Overmedicating can be unintentional. In these situations, a nurse overloaded with tasks to perform might administer the wrong dosage of medications. Rowles and High (2003: 186) detail a situation where a woman monitoring her husband's care unearthed an overmedication situation:

He was agitated. The third shift called the doctor at 4 a.m., and he was still out that afternoon when we arrived. My son and I took him to the bathroom, and, honey, he was just like somebody drugged. He couldn't put one foot over the other. Al is a small man, you know what I mean. He doesn't need a lot of medication. They overmedicated in giving him something that, you know, what they give a 200-pound man.

Along with medication issues, medical dereliction also involves staff failing to turn the bodies of bedridden residents. When medical conditions confine older people with frail skin to their beds, there is a high possibility that a decubitus ulcer, better known as a bedsore, can form. If these painful, open wounds become infected, they can lead to serious cases of gangrene. We know from firsthand experience that the possibility of the infected area needing amputation increases if a bedsore reaches this point.

Bureaucratic Backwardness

We define personal negligence as staff failing to provide sufficient upkeep of tangible features of residents. This includes clothing and personal hygiene. With our content analysis, 134 references to personal negligence appear, making up 26.7 percent of the physical maltreatment rituals analyzed.

Accounts show busy aides often fail to properly clean or clothe residents. A former aide told us:

> [The clothing and hygiene issue] was the most noticeable problem with staff efficiency. We rarely had the staff needed to spend time with each resident in the morning. There was always tension between the third shift and the morning shift regarding how many residents were up and ready for the day. I was lectured on several occasions about being too slow and leaving too many residents for the first shift to

get ready. Sometimes aides came into the rooms, lifted the residents into chairs with slippers and a blanket and rolled them out to the lobby. I would often see residents without their hair combed or their face washed properly.

Mollette (2001) says he visited the nursing home his wife was in many times, seeing residents who had gone days without baths, having their hair combed, or teeth brushed. As a former activity director, Poxon (2004) explains her frustrations of having residents attend recreational events with large amounts of feces accumulated under their nails. Deutschman (2005) tells of residents wearing the same clothes from Monday to Friday. Laird (1979: 99) elaborates on the clothing issue stating, "Florence had a daffodil-yellow dress which didn't entirely satisfy her. One day she said, 'I believe I'll give this to Annie. The color will be becoming to her ... ' Annie wore it. But to our disappointment, the aide had put it on her backwards." It would be easy to assume that putting on a dress backwards is a mistake and not intentional ritualistic personal negligence. Employees, as with the medical dereliction example, have full plates and slip up. However, putting clothes on the wrong way is often an unfortunate case of intentional bureaucratic backwardness. Kayser-Jones (1981: 46) explains:

> Many residents at Pacific Manor do not have personal clothing, and what is provided for them is ill-fitting, un-pressed, and inappropriate. The available clothing (contributed by charitable organizations or left behind by previous patients) is stuffed in large cardboard boxes; no attempt is made to keep it neat or pressed. When someone needs a shirt or dress, attendants pull out whatever they can find; if the appropriate piece of attire is not available, a substitute is made. Mrs. White, an attractive 78-year-old woman who normally sat in a wheelchair clad in a sweater and slip, had to wear a bathrobe tied backwards around her waist to simulate a skirt when the therapist came to help her walk. To lack underclothes or to have clothes put

on backwards is also dehumanizing for the elderly. Robes often are put on this way, staff informed me, to decrease the amount of work involved in changing an incontinent patient and to decrease the amount of laundry. If robes are put on backwards and not tucked under, they are not soiled when patients are incontinent.

With so much to do, the emphasis on hygienic care is not what it should be either. Levels of hygiene people outside of nursing home walls might find repugnant are viewed as normal by nursing home employees. With hygienic care carrying a prime value, aides have the ability to withhold it as punishment when residents upset them. Shield (1988: 159) states, "Staff retribution can result when residents are too demanding. In subtle and not so subtle ways, staff members neglect or delay doing things."

Ecological Oversight

We define environmental negligence as staff members failing to maintain domains of interaction such as living areas, recreational rooms, kitchens, and grounds outside of the facility. This includes aspects of cleanliness that have the potential to put nursing home residents in health-related danger. With our content analysis, there are 117 references to actions involving environmental negligence, making up 23.3 percent of the physical maltreatment rituals analyzed. Gubrium (1993: 170) details one account provided by a former nursing home surveyor turned resident:

> I think that cleanliness is a problem. I think here roaches are a problem. We are having a roach war here, okay? They are trying to kill the roaches. I myself am not a roach person. I don't like them. I used to write out nursing homes for roaches all over. And this place has probably got as good roaches as I have ever run into.... I mean, I was sitting with Harry [another resident] last night talking and one of them walks up the back of my dresser. I do not keep loose food in

my room, okay? An experienced surveyor knows this. We have got a really, truly serious, bad roach problem.

The issue is not that nursing homes directly cause physical harm to residents by not maintaining a clean environment, but their ecological oversight has the potential to increase the likelihood that disease-related germs, which can have a physical impact, spread among residents. Previously mentioned interviewee Billy Hill explains his concerns:

> When my Mom had an infection, she was moved to the nursing home's isolation wing. When isolation wing aides cleaned Mom after she defecated, they would then toss the feces-covered rags into an open box in Mom's room and leave them there all day. Often when I came in the evening, flies would be buzzing about the opened box, and the stench was overwhelming. I reported this deplorable practice to the isolation wing nurse, who explained that they only pick up the trash from isolation wing residents once a day. I found that an inadequate explanation, so I then spoke to the chief administrator; he was responsive and made sure this unsanitary practice stopped. However, my assumption is that this practice continued for other isolation wing residents, for there was probably no one to intervene on their behalf.

In his seminal research on nursing homes in the 1960s, Henry (1963) argues employees ignore potential health risks when not adequately cleaning standard items in resident rooms, such as bedpans left dirty and dried with feces at bedsides. More than forty years later, Billy's comments confirm that not much has changed.

Don't Trust People in White

We define bodily harm as any physical abuse by nursing home employees directed toward residents. This includes anything from the misuse of physical restraints to acts akin to assault and battery. One hundred and seven references to bodily harm appear in the content analysis portion of this research, comprising 21.3 percent of the physical maltreatment rituals studied.

In terms of bureaucratic connections discussed in Chapter 4, Stannard (1973) suggests sometimes staff give scalding hot baths to residents to punish them for creating problems. In what we interpret as another form of punishment, employees sometimes improperly use physical restraints on residents who disrupt work-flow. Paterniti (2000: 106) provides an account:

> Out of frustration and a perceived need to keep Scott restrained, aides frequently tied a square knot in the nylon vest restraint that secured Scott in a reclining Gerry chair (geriatric chairs used to create less pressure on parts of the body). Some even remarked, "If you're a mechanic, let's see you get yourself out of this one!" On one occasion, an aide locked Scott, tied to a chair, in the janitors' closet. The aide entertained himself by keeping records of how long it took Scott to work his way out of the restraints and to the door of the closet. Ironically, additional work to this staff member's schedule, generated under his own control, seemed to present no obstacle to his work timetable.

The misuse of restraints is also a ritual response to understaffing. Diamond (1992: 182) explains:

> Mary Ryan, like many others, spent all day in the dayroom, secured to her chair with a restraining vest. "How y' doin' today, Mary?" I once asked in passing. She answered the question with a question. "Why do I have to sit here with this thing on?" I responded auto-matically with the trained answer, "That's so you won't fall. You know that." "Oh, get away from me," she reacted with disgust. "I don't trust anybody in white anymore." Stunned by her rejection,

and not completely confident of my own answer, I passed the question on to Beulah Feders, the LPN in charge. "Beulah, why does she have to wear that thing all the time?" Beulah accompanied her quick comeback with a chuckle. "That's so they don't have to hire any more of you."

Sometimes residents act out violently against staff and the nursing home has to restrain them to protect themselves and other residents. The senior author got his first taste of this on his first day working in a nursing home in the late 1990s. The executive director was showing him around when she displayed her lack of knowledge on the condition of a resident. In an attempt to show how close she was to her residents, she leaned down to a sweet looking old woman and yelled in her ear, "How are you doing?" The resident, who she did not know had a history of violence, pulled her arm back like a major league baseball pitcher and swung an opened hand to the director's face. After the fierce impact, it was clear the director was not pleased. She mumbled a few orders to the nurse aide standing nearby. Restraints were surely in the unruly resident's future. The director did not make any more false-hearted attempts at friendliness on our tour.

Unfortunately, some employees do not resort to restraints when assaulted, but simply carry out the same action against the resident. Tisdale's conversation with a staff member explains one worker's opinion on bodily harm, "Some are kind, some are cruel. They kick me, I kick them" (1987: 109). This reveals a dynamic of reciprocity in terms of abuse. However, not all staff members have the same perspective on bodily harm. Shield (1988: 76) explains the attitude of one physical therapist:

> She is telling me about the time one of the residents came to physical therapy and had a bruise that, to the physical therapist, looked

suspicious. She was sticking her neck out, she knew, by reporting it, but she decided to act. She phoned the charge nurse on the resident's floor and reported it. She also wrote it up. Though she knew she was inviting employee resentment and anger by her actions, she felt it was important to be a resident's advocate and agent for change in this way. She was letting employees on the floor know she was not going to avoid difficult issues and help cover things up.

We believe lower-level employees of nursing homes, such as aides, sometimes normalize neglect and abuse. Since they are the ones who see the most of it in their everyday work, they sometimes will deem it acceptable and a functional part of their job. We think administrators are aware of neglect and abuse, but since they do not perform hands-on care and do not have to deal with residents as much as other employees they can repress its presence. However, physical therapists are in a different hierarchical position. We do not see them as administrative staff, and they certainly are not floor staff either. Some are not even housed in nursing homes, but just show up at scheduled times for therapy. This isolates them from the bureaucratic rituals that facilitate maltreatment and, as in the case above, provides them the psychological freedom to reject abuse and neglect as normal parts of elder care. We also believe physical therapists are the least likely of nursing home employees to objectify residents, which would explain their compassionate perspectives on maltreatment.

Physical therapists promote rehabilitation and independence while other aspects of nursing home life downplay them. Residents know this and many report that it boosts their psychological well-being to see the physical therapist. As Shield (1988) explains, the physical therapy room is a unique place within the nursing home and has a different atmosphere. When residents are there they joke, smile, laugh, and flirt. Hale (2005: 181) explains that the "closest relationships Mother developed were with the head therapist and the therapist's aides."

As with other aspects of neglect and abuse discussed in this book, bodily harm is not always intentional. It can be the unintentional byproduct of bureaucratic demands. Here, issues of efficiency and the constraints of understaffing are relevant. An aide explained to us:

> One night we were very short staffed and I was asked to go up on the isolated hall alone. I was told by another aide that had worked there for years that I was supposed to get certain residents up and ready by myself in the morning. If these residents were not ready, the morning aides would put in a complaint. One of the residents that I was told to get up was supposed to have two people assisting, but this aide said that one person could easily get him up. The resident fell over while he was sitting on the bed and I was attempting to get him dressed. He was too heavy for me to catch and he hit his head on the bed board. He had a small cut on his forehead, but he didn't hit it very hard. It took ten minutes for someone to come and assist me, but I didn't want to leave the resident alone. A few days later, I was brought into the administrator's office and reprimanded for attempting to move the resident by myself. I expressed my concern about being alone on an isolated hall with so many residents, but I didn't feel that my concerns were taken seriously.

Architectural Matters

After our content analysis started, we saw themes related to physical issues and architectural matters emerging. This is another of our "other" classifications, so we did not include it in our total numbers for physical maltreatment, especially since it does not have a direct link to bureaucratic culture. However, we still want to note its relevance to nursing home care.

Sources from our content analysis and data from our interviews indicate that the design of many nursing homes creates problems. For example, consider room size. Even able-bodied residents sometimes cannot navigate small rooms. They end up bumping into shelves or nightstands, which results in bodily harm. Room size also causes problems for employees. Gass (2004: 93–94) explains the work limitations caused by the size of resident rooms:

> We roll into her room, I reach over her shoulder to open the bathroom door ahead of us then swing my foot behind to kick the outer door closed. Entry door, bathroom door, and closet door in every room clash against each other in an architectural feud of door clanging, gouged wood veneers, and scarred varnish. The owners built five nursing homes previous to this one. I joke to Marge that they needed a lot of practice to get the architecture this wrong.

Organizational Variation

Concerning rituals of physical maltreatment in our content analysis data, we have high frequencies of medical dereliction and personal negligence. The accounts we examined foster the impression that nursing home employees both intentionally and unintentionally engage in these harmful ritualized practices. The high level of salience of these rituals reflected in the multiple examples presented here illustrates the perceived importance of medical dereliction and personal negligence, especially when bureaucratic demands require minimal work disruptions. Comment on ownership variation in these two categories of physical mishandling is also relevant. An overwhelming number, around 70 percent in both categories, came from for-profit sources.

We found fewer instances of environmental negligence and bodily harm rituals, but they appear just as troubling as the other two categories. However, we do not believe a high level of salience exists in the environmental negligence category. Rituals promoting poor environmental conditions are not intentional and are certainly not issues holding great weight in the minds of nursing home employees. Bodily harm rituals do appear salient as seen in a number of striking examples involving the intentional misuse of restraints and unintentional injury caused by bureaucratic pressure. As with the first two categories, we also found around 70 percent of references to environmental negligence and bodily harm in for-profit sources.

The American humorist Evan Esar once said that zoos are "an excellent place to study the habits of human beings" (Baxter 2008: 96). As this chapter sadly indicates, whether it is intentional or not, nursing homes are an excellent place to see people treated as if they live in a zoo. It also makes us wonder: Is life better for the animals in the zoo? We stated earlier in this chapter that you do not hear about residents mauling visitors. If the elder care catastrophe keeps on pace, we are sure to hear those stories soon enough.

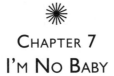

Chapter 7
I'm No Baby

The tongue like a sharp knife ... kills without
drawing blood.

Buddha

Centuries ago, a prince facing a future framed by riches and power
decided to break out of his sheltered existence and see the world.
Worried about his son's well-being, his father did not want him to
go. So the prince's father sent guards to travel ahead of the twenty-
something prince on each trip he took. Their objective was clear:
Make sure the prince did not encounter anything that would affect
his destiny as heir to the throne. The guards succeeded in keeping
the prince from physical harm, but they could do little to keep his
worldviews intact once he experienced what people call the "Four
Passing Sights" (Smith 1992).

On his first trip, the prince saw an old man with visible physical
deterioration. Leaning on a staff, the man could barely stand he was
shaking so badly. The prince had never thought about aging until
that moment. On his second trip, the prince encountered a disease-
ridden man lying by the road. The prince had never thought about

the impact of sickness before. On his third trip, he saw a corpse. Until then, he had never acknowledged that death is inevitable. On his fourth and final trip, he saw a poor monk, draped in rags and with a look on his face of serenity, reflecting an extreme form of happiness. Thus the prince came to realize the physical realities of age, sickness, and death. He also came to believe that true happiness is not something obtainable in the physical world, but something found through spiritual enlightenment. The prince later became one of the most important religious figures in the world—Buddha (Mehrotra, Wagner, and Fried 2009).

Aside from providing the world with some interesting ideas on aging and death, Buddha provided insight in a variety of areas. This includes the acknowledgement, represented by the quote opening this chapter, that sticks and stones may break bones, but words can be just as harmful. Here, we analyze the link between bureaucracy and verbal abuse of nursing home residents.

Verbal Abuse in Nursing Home Care

As Table 7.1 illustrates, 346 ritualized acts of verbal abuse appear in the content analysis portion of our research. They include aspects of infantilization, spoken aggression, and ignoring.

Table 7.1 Frequencies for Verbal Abuse Rituals

Subdivision	Number	Percent
Infantilization	148	42.8
Spoken aggression	100	28.9
Ignoring	98	28.3
Total	346	100.0

Geriatrics or Pediatrics

We define infantilization as speaking in a condescending way that reduces the status of a resident to that of a young child. Infantilization as a form of elder mistreatment is an emerging area of concern for researchers (for more, see Gresham 2007). They believe infantilization is more widespread and harmful than many people involved with elder care would like to believe. Gass (2004: 88) was discussing this issue with a neurologist, who indicated to him that when you are dealing with adults losing control over their bodies, "geriatrics becomes pediatrics." Is that the appropriate attitude needed for quality elder care? Some researchers do not think so. They believe caregivers need to be more attuned to the subtle nuances of communication that degrade the status of the old by treating them like children, whether it is in adult day cares (Salari 2006), dentists' offices (Dolinsky and Dolinsky 2008), or in the case of our research, nursing homes. With our content analysis, 148 references to infantilization appear, making up 42.8 percent of the verbal abuse rituals studied. Kayser-Jones (1981: 39) provides a solid representation:

> At Pacific Manor there were innumerable incidents of staff treating the residents like children. Authoritarian scoldings of the aged by staff were common. For example, one day a nurse aide walked into the lounge and, seeing a puddle of water on the floor, asked loudly, "Who wet the floor?" Pointing her finger at one woman, she inquired in an accusing voice, "Did you wet the floor?" Very embarrassed at being singled out as the culprit, the patient replied, "Why, no it wasn't me." Staff frequently command patients in a parental voice: "Shut up," "Stay in your chair," "Go to your place for lunch," "I want you to go in and put on a dress, now get dressed," and "Sit down, Grace." Such commands are often accompanied by gestures,

such as pointing a finger at the aged person, forcibly taking him by the arm, or "leading" him to a chair.

Of course staff members do not always intend to be outright malicious with infantilizing comments. Diamond (1992: 138) points out:

> She was using the term "baby" to ridicule the rule, which many residents made fun of as well, that bibs had to be tied on to each resident for each meal. "Baby" was often used, and in more than one way. In some contexts it was used to create fictive family roles. Dorothy Tomason put her arm around Joanne Macon when she cried. "C'mere, my baby, now what's the trouble." "Baby" was also used more broadly as a designation of the impersonal, referring to infants who were incompetent and unaware. "Oh, you work up there on the baby floor," observed a first-floor nursing assistant. Another advised, "Oh, don't worry about these people; when they get old they all start acting just like babies."

Clearly, infantilization takes different forms. Nursing home employees use it to ridicule institutional rules that breed infantilization (though we believe this reinforces and reproduces the very act they are trying to ridicule). They also use it as a form of cognitive resonance. They are providing the type of parental care given to infants, such as bathing and feeding, but doing it for an adult. We believe that for their caregiving to make more sense to them, they rely on previous relationship structures such as parent–child relationships because it eases subconscious confusion to refer to the adults they are working with as children. Finally, nursing home employees use infantilization as a form of objectification.

We think that when nursing home employees do not view residents as adults, it is easier to view them as objects of labor and subsequently easier to deflect emotional components of care.

Ironically, a historical connection between infants and objectification exists. Before the 1400s, the concept of childhood did not even exist. It only developed after medicine and technological advancements allowed a majority of children to live past the first few years of life. Parents would not treat infants as human because they did not want a strong emotional attachment knowing the likelihood of an infant's survival was slim (Bernard 1992). With nursing home care, perhaps we are seeing the same trend play out, except at the other end of the life cycle.

Regional variation in speech is also relevant. Savishinsky (1991: 75) points out that in the facility he observed there was an "infantilizing habit of addressing residents with unearned terms of endearment: 'honey,' 'love,' 'sweetie,' and 'dear' were patronizing to the ear." Our research did not consider separating sources written about southern nursing homes from others, but it is important to note that in some areas of the southern United States people use terms like "baby" when engaging in everyday interaction regardless of age. In relation to the unintentional use of infantilizing words, you could argue that most people in the South do not use these phrases for literal interpretation. We know in these instances staff cannot control how others interpret their language, but we think nursing home employees should realize that not every resident interprets infantilizing language as endearing, even in southern nursing homes. Moreover, when staff freely infantilize language without malicious intent, it has the potential to do the most damage, especially when directed toward older individuals already susceptible to poor self-image due to the conditions of dependency and functional impairment (see Whitmer and Whitbourne 1997).

The spoken word is not the only thing producing ritualized infantilization in nursing homes. Aside from requirements on assisted bathing and eating, other infantilizing actions exist. Some are required, such as the use of "adult diapers" for incontinent residents. However, many are not. Consider having Santa Claus come to give out presents on Christmas (Metz 1999), or various aspects of television viewing. We know of employees putting on cartoons for residents to watch on television and borrowing kid movies from local day cares to show residents. When mix-ups happen and children's shows are not on the viewing menu, staff become disturbed since many do not see adult television as appropriate, even if it is adults who will be watching. Poxon (2004: 66–67) notes:

> Barry volunteered to tape movies for us from HBO for our movie matinee. He was taping Beethoven 2 for us to show the next day. He fell asleep during the taping and the next morning he rewound the video and brought it with him to work. When it was time for the movie, my assistant Geneva, put in the movie and went to the nurses' station to do some charting. After an hour or so she was approached by one of the nurses who asked her what type of movie she was showing the residents. So she went into the TV room to find several nurses and residents watching an adult X-rated movie. Geneva immediately stopped the video. One of our residents who was engrossed in what was on the screen hollered, "Why did you turn that off? I was enjoying that." What had happened was after Barry went to sleep an adult movie came on. Since he didn't have the time to view it before bringing it in he was totally unaware of all he had taped.

In terms of power, the inability to control your own television viewing is quite demoralizing. Kidder (1993: 203–204) illustrates this situation with the story of Earl, who liked to watch shows knowing his wife was at home watching the same thing:

> Sometimes Earl's roommate got confused, and the man was prey to those abrupt fits of weeping that strokes often induce. Once, over a month ago, he had been parked out by the nurses' station and had

started weeping saying he couldn't watch what he wanted on TV. But that had all been straightened out, Earl thought. Earl had asked his roommate, "Mind if I watch this show?" His roommate had said he didn't mind. As always, he had reminded Jean to be sure and watch this show at home tonight. Suddenly, two young women entered. One of them picked up the remote control from Earl's bedside table. She put it down on his roommate's table and said, "Mr. Duncan, you can't have this." But Earl's roommate himself had given Earl the control to handle. "*Mister* Duncan," said the other young woman, "you *cannot* have that." Earl was not a wrathful man. When the social worker visited him the next morning, he simply asked her how many days' notice one had to give before leaving Linda Manor. Earl told her that he felt as though he'd been treated like a five-year-old.

Aware of infantilizing rituals, residents acknowledge it as a problem for their image maintenance. Diamond (1992:138) explains:

Bedridden Frances Wasserman protested, "Just 'cause I have to lay here in this gown doesn't mean I'm a baby." The same protests came up at meal time in the same tone, in part, because of bibs but also for the reason expressed by Mrs. Herman, who was blind. "You know, I was a field nurse, too. I'm no baby just because someone has to help me eat."

Some aides are aware of the disenchantment of care that infantilization creates for residents and refuse to use infantilizing language. In one of our interviews for this book, a former aide noted, "On my first training day I witnessed the aide that I was shadowing pinch the cheeks of a resident and treat her like she was a baby." She went on to explain that by the time she worked in the facility for several months she had "heard several of the staff use a baby voice when talking to some of the residents." Displaying her displeasure with the practice, she went on to state, "I never felt comfortable [infantilizing] people in this manner."

Residents contribute to infantilization as well. We have heard residents talk to each other with baby talk and even request dolls or "security" blankets for themselves. We believe that this self-imposed infantilization assists in the progression of dependency on staff. Knowing that employees view them as helpless, needy, and infantile, residents will sometimes demand services when they could act on their own. Gass (2004: 171) explains his feeling on this issue when working as an aide by stating, "Maybe if I treat these people like responsible adults, they may begin to treat us a bit more reasonably and maybe respect themselves a tiny bit more in the process."

Shut Up and Eat

We define spoken aggression as the hostile launching of vocal attacks by staff directed against a resident. In our content analysis, 100 references to it appear, making up 28.9 percent of the verbal abuse rituals analyzed. Many of the sources indicate that spoken aggression is used to deter residents from annoying staff. Howsden (1981: 76) explains:

> A typical encounter includes a complaint of a headache, stomach ache, or another patient who has caused them distress. The patient is not ignored, but merely put off with the typical response, "Oh, go sit down and you will feel better," or "You ... go find something to do like feeding the cat," or "Go help Mrs. C. with her chair." The tactic is one of diversion, which, if unsuccessful, is followed by threats, such as "If you don't leave me alone, I'll send you to your room."

Administrative staff also sometimes show favor to nurses and aides who use spoken aggression because it speeds up the completion of work tasks. Speaking to residents in an intimidating tone cuts back on their resistance and demands for service. In data from one of our interviews, an aide comments on herself and another aide trying to get a resident to comply with their demands. The co-worker called the resident a "mean old woman" to her face while they were struggling with her "combative" actions. We find it interesting that nursing home employees sometimes use war-related adjectives to describe residents. Regardless, the interviewee did not clarify whether administrators encouraged such speech patterns, but in one of our content analysis sources, administration clearly praised an aide who verbally assaulted patients to gain their compliance. Foner (1992: 61) explains:

> When the woman complained that she could not eat because her foot hurt, Ms. James screamed, "Shut up you and eat you. Eat. You think I have all day for you." And she turned to another woman, "You're such a nasty pig. You hear me, drink." When a resident Ms. James had put on the toilet complained, she barked, "Sit there. Just sit. I don't care what hurts, just sit there. Sit down; don't bother me about being ready." As the LPN passed, Ms. James loudly commented so that the residents could hear: "Two dingbats I got here. One has shit coming out of her ass and the other one says her back hurts." Ms. James humiliated and verbally abused patients out in the open: in front of nurses, administrators, doctors, and visitors. Yet she received the best evaluation on the floor and was given privileges denied to other aides.

Finally, another technique involves the escalation of verbal assaults to threatening language. Data we collected from a man whose mother is in a nursing home in the foothills of the Ozark Mountains reflects this theme. The facility has good marks from the state survey team. On their most recent inspection, inspectors gave them four out of five stars on health issues. However, they received only two out of five stars for their nursing and aide staff rating. This means that they are below average on the number of nurses and aides they have per resident. We speculate this under-staffing puts the nurses and aides in the facility under high levels of pressure, which sometimes makes them resort to threatening residents to keep their request for services at bay. With respect to requests for help, the interviewee stated, "Mom has reported to me an instance in which one of the aides yelled at her for pressing her call button twice in succession … another aide said she was going to beat [her] up … another aide has told her that she was going to be thrown out of the nursing home."

Failing to Respond Is a Response

We define ignoring as nursing home employees refusing to take notice of communication initiated by residents. This includes ig-noring attempts at conversation or disregarding audible requests for personal and medical assistance. With ignoring, we believe employees are not actively engaging in verbal abuse, but pas-sively engaging in it by refusing to communicate at all. In other words, failing to respond is a conscious, decision-based response to people in need. This is distinct from personal negligence and medical dereliction discussed in Chapter 6. With those RSPs, nursing home staff recognize personal and medical issues, but fail to do anything about them. In this case, residents make personal or medical requests without staff acknowledgement. Ninety-eight references to ignoring appear in the content analysis portion of this research, comprising 28.3 percent of the verbal maltreatment rituals studied.

With regard to bureaucratic constraints, we once again see ignoring as a maltreatment pattern based on residents disrupting goals of efficiency in a workday. Paterniti (2000: 106) explains that nursing home employees tend to residents whom they identify as disruptive or incompetent when they feel like it because most residents who request assistance do not have pressing needs. Nursing staff have to ignore them for the sake of completing important work, even if the nursing home limits the opportunities for residents to engage in activities to keep pain off their minds. Gass (2004: 70) elaborates on this dynamic, arguing that the longer he worked in a nursing home as an aide, the more he realized he could not help everyone:

> It is not unusual to walk down a back hall and see half a dozen residents trapped in their wheelchairs, arms flailing, moaning, begging desperately for help. Nothing seems to breed impatience like a complete lack of agenda. Our residents have nothing to do but focus on their pain. At times our halls become a veritable sea of moaning, crying, begging, and whimpering. It is simply not possible to alleviate the waves of pain, anger, anxiety, boredom, despair, and loneliness. If I have learned anything from coping with this work, it is the need to say no. Before this job, I would not have thought myself capable of hearing a helpless old lady beg for my attention and keep right on walking without breaking my stride. But now I do. I do it every day.

Reflecting on patterns of ignoring, one resident told Gubrium (1993: 144), "You ask them to do something and they ignore you like dirty shit." Mollette (2001: 58) observed aides shutting doors so they would not have to "hear what they are being asked to do" by residents. From earlier work, Gubrium (1975) explains that residents have various resources, including being uncooperative or complaining, to influence work patterns of lower staff. Employees working the floor know the residents who tend to be uncooperative or complain, and failing to acknowledge those residents sends a message to others that they should not disrupt organizational tasks or they will suffer the same fate. As discussed in Chapter 6, residents comply because they fear being stigmatized as a troublemaker. However, this does not keep residents, and even other staff, from complaining to family members about nursing home employees ignoring them. Reflecting the issue of staff separation discussed in Chapter 4, Mollette (2001: 64–66) details his wife's and a former aide's grievances with a male nurse named Max:

> "Glenn, when Max comes in here and I ask him to turn me over he simply ignores me and walks right back out the door." "Glenn, she's telling you the truth," chimed in [her roommate]. "He just walks right out the door." I would later find out from an aide that Max did this all the time not only to Karen but also other [residents] who needed him. He was the only nurse working third shift and he was all that the patients on Karen's wing had. An aide who quit … told me, "Glenn, I caught Max several times turning on Karen's call light and walking out of the room. Instead of him staying in the room and doing whatever she was asking him to do, he would turn on the call light and leave it for an aide to do."

Vaughan (1999) argues that routine practices in organizations can have unintended consequences. When repeatedly performing a task, it frequently becomes second nature, even if it harms others. Nurses and aides, especially those dealing with understaffing, ritualistically ignore residents. As earlier comments by Gass (2004) indicate, the nursing home culture normalizes it as acceptable. However, not all nursing home employees feel comfortable with deciding who to ignore and who not to ignore. As one former aide told us, "We always answered the call lights, but sometimes there was one person on a hall and several lights on at the same time. In those cases, we had to make decisions on who needed help first." Even if we think it is catastrophic that ritualized ignoring takes place in nursing homes, we acknowledge that having to make split-second decisions on who deserves help over others cannot be a pleasant chore, especially when it has horrifying results. Paterniti (2000: 106) explains:

> This afternoon, I talked with a staff member over lunch about some of the residents at Merimore who had died during my days off. Jessica said, "It was during lunch, ya know, when we're real busy. As usual, we were still passing trays, and Hazel put on her [nurse call] light. Naturally, Michele [Hazel's usual aide] just ignored it." Jessica noted with a certain matter-of-factness: Anyone who had any knowledge of Hazel, her deficiencies, and the work routine would have, of course, followed the same course of action. She continued, "When Michele went in [to Hazel's room] to pick up Hazel's tray, she [Hazel] didn't respond. She wasn't breathing. Hazel was dead."

Organizational Variation

With respect to rituals of verbal abuse in our content analysis data, the greatest number of references are in the infantilization category. Nearly all of the examples create the impression that infantilization is a salient part of nursing home culture. Fewer references to spoken aggression and ignoring lead us to believe that they are not as problematic. Spoken aggression examples do not create the impression that employees see aggressive verbal assaults as an essential part of work, but salient examples of ignoring give the impression that employees view overlooking resident requests for conversation and care as a necessity. With infantilization, we did find 57 percent of references in for-profit sources and only 43 percent in nonprofit sources. The percentages of spoken aggression and ignoring references were close to even in for-profit and nonprofit sources.

We wonder what Buddha would think of the modern-day nursing home. What would it be like if he were alive today and living in an elder care facility? Would he sit in his room turning to meditation in order to block out his physical suffering? Would nurses and aides tell him he looked like a big baby with his bald head and spiritual grin while turning his television to the Cartoon Network? Would they respect his practice of limiting himself to just a few drops of food a day, or yell at him with demands to eat more of his food? And if he pushed his call light, would anyone come?

CHAPTER 8
ALTERNATIVES TO BUREAUCRACY
IN NURSING HOMES

> Once fully established, bureaucracy is among
> those social structures which are the hardest to
> destroy.
>
> Max Weber

In the previous chapters, we present a typology for nursing home resident maltreatment. We detail aspects of emotional neglect, physical maltreatment, and verbal abuse. We provide future researchers with a way to classify neglect and abuse in nursing homes, and we legitimize arguments that a bureaucratic organizational culture facilitates poor levels of care. However, we want to reiterate that we do not think most people who work in nursing homes premeditate most of the harm caused to residents. In our minds, nursing home employees are living in what Max Weber's work discusses as an "iron cage." Even those with the best intentions must bend to the will of hierarchical divisions, rules, documentation, and efficiency. Bureaucratic institutional logics place a stranglehold on nursing homes, shaping their goals and the ways that people think in them, for better or worse.

As we argue in Chapter 2, rituals, which we identify as RSPs, are crucial to the understanding everyday life in nursing homes. RSPs—repeated actions with symbolic significance—help form ways of thinking in organizations and set the tone for specific patterns of behavior. If the predominant pattern of rituals in nursing homes revolves around the idea of bureaucracy, a majority of people's thoughts and behaviors in the nursing home context will involve bureaucratic themes. However, different kinds of ritualized practices that are not necessarily bureaucratic in nature can exist in organizations, and we believe the injection of alternative RSPs in nursing homes can enhance people's lives, empower individuals, and build close social ties and a sense of community. Though Max Weber (1946) argued that established bureaucracy is impossible to destroy, we believe that the introduction of alternative RSPs, implemented in a serious and systematic way, has the potential to create change in nursing homes. Others present a similar argument in a movement identified as "culture change." In this chapter, we briefly review the culture change movement. We also detail aspects of an alternative ritual model we developed that directly relates to culture change themes.

The Culture Change Movement

The movement toward culture change in nursing homes involves a shift away from the traditional nursing home model. It argues that anything employees, families, and residents can do to increase resident autonomy and control, known as resident-centered care, has the ability to change nursing homes in a positive way. As Elizabeth Brawley, of the American Society on Aging, notes, "Successfully implementing culture change can transform a facility into a home, a patient into a person, and a schedule into a choice" (2007: 9). The culture change movement includes several identifiable segments: the Pioneer Network, the Eden Alternative, the Green House Initiative, and the Wellspring model.

The Pioneer Network is a group of researchers and elder care providers who advocate general principles they believe have the potential to better the lives of residents. They include a desire for employees to know each person in the facility, recognizing that each person can make a difference in improving facility conditions, and that quality relationships are the building block of culture change. Pioneer themes also focus on spirituality, risk-taking if it enhances quality of life, and putting people before employment tasks (Lustbader 2000).

Physician Bill Thomas created the Eden Alternative in 1991. He and his supporters advocate that there should be less bureaucracy in nursing homes. Measures in the Eden Alternative ideology focus on reducing symptoms of loneliness, helplessness, and boredom, which Thomas believes account for the majority of misery for residents. Additional measures include taking steps to promote resident roles in providing care, facilitating the likelihood of unpredictable interaction patterns, and downplaying medical orientations in elder care. The Eden Alternative also argues for the injection of plants, animal life (such as pets), and children into elder care environments, implying that the presence of these things creates a more humane habitat (Thomas 1996). Research indicates the Eden Alternative not only reduces the use of antidepressants, the number of bedsores, and the use of physical restraints among nursing home residents, but also lowers staff absenteeism levels (Brawley and Kleyman 2007).

The Green House Initiative is also the brainchild of Thomas. Green houses are small, residential buildings that exist in clusters.

The clusters represent a nursing home. Each home-like building has up to 10 people living in it. Living areas have private bedrooms and bathrooms. Two certified nursing assistants (CNAs) with advanced training, called Shahbazim, are on duty at each cluster. They act less like the dispensers of medical care and more like home health aides. No nurses' stations exist. When residents need doctors and other specialized medical staff, aides call them to the facility. Research indicates that residents in green houses experience less of a decline in ADLs, less incontinence, less depression, and reduced antipsychotic drug use. It also shows that nursing home employees in the green house model have closer, quality relationships with residents in addition to a higher level of job satisfaction (Niesz 2005).

A conglomerate of eleven nonprofit nursing homes in Wisconsin developed the Wellspring model. The facilities decided to alter their organizational culture with core ideas used to advance better care. Elements of the Wellspring model include making sure upper-level employees are dedicated to resident care above all else and developing interdisciplinary care teams to train employees. Employees within each department in the nursing home, as well as across all departments in the conglomerate, are encouraged to have open lines of communication in order to fight the likelihood of staff separation conflict and increase communication among staff. The Wellspring model also implements a geriatric nurse practitioner program. In this program, nurse practitioners in the consortium train employees on specific clinical guidelines relating to physical well-being, incontinence issues, skin care, nutrition, and resident behavior management. Wellspring also calls for a greater recognition of problems experienced by the "front-line" staff: CNAs. It empowers CNAs by pulling them into decision-making processes as much as possible (Reinhard and Stone 2001).

The Centralized Alternative Ritual Enactment (CARE) Model

With the hope that the culture change movement can have a positive effect on nursing homes, we propose several recommendations based on our research. Many are person-centered and direct attention to everyone in the organization, including residents *and* employees. We call our collection of recommendations the "Centralized Alternative Ritual Enactment" (CARE) model. The CARE model refers to alternative ritual enactments being centralized in the sense that they have a particular focus; that is, developing alternative nonbureaucratic (more humane) rituals. Although the ultimate focus is on the ritual behaviors of people, these proposals also address the organizational rules, arrangements, situational pressures, and other social factors that facilitate both bureaucratic and alternative RSPs. Our recommendations relate to the theoretical premise of *transformative structural ritualization* (Knottnerus 1997). It indicates that the more dominant or important new ritualized behaviors are, the greater is their potential to change thoughts and patterns of behavior in social contexts. Reflecting and extending lines of thought in the culture change movement, we believe alternative rituals have the ability to move nursing home care closer to what it should be, as opposed to what bureaucratic rituals have made it.

Some of our recommendations are nonspecific and relate to the general orientation of staff and residents to issues of bureaucracy. Others involve specific recommendations that administrators and other employees could implement to replace or counteract the negative effects of bureaucracy and its facilitation of emotional, physical, and verbal neglect and abuse. Most of these involve alternative rituals and different techniques that practitioners could implement in order to reduce, if not eliminate, different forms of abuse. The steps identified here involve both big and small changes in policy and procedures. Of course, we would stress that what might appear to some to be a small change can be of profound importance for residents and their daily experiences in nursing homes. We should note that our recommendations might overlap to some degree. In addition, they may resemble other ideas in the culture change movement, but we discuss them in a slightly different way since they directly relate to the research in this book. Regardless, because we believe that all of them are important, we formally highlight each one so readers can easily identify, appreciate, and, depending on the reader, implement them.

Downplay bureaucracy. The industry could work with policy makers to either cut back on or revise regulations. For example, sometimes it might be beneficial to accept health risks to promote quality of life. This could involve emphasizing the emotional side of care and not the bureaucratic. In other words, strictly enforced rules that promote dependency for medical reasons should not be a focus. We should reward staff for building personal relationships with residents and not for task efficiency. This does not just have to involve nurses and their support staff. Research indicates that when CNAs receive a higher number of rewards for good care, the less likely are residents to experience bedsores. Moreover, facilities with a low number of resident bedsores have lower turnover rates (Barry, Brannon, and Mor 2005). Nursing homes could even encourage non-direct-care staff such as housekeepers to spend small bits of extra time with residents and even evaluate their performance not just based on cleaning tasks but on positive interaction with residents as well.

In addition, even state guidelines that generate bureaucratic demands should include measures concerned with emotional care and the quality of life of residents. They should still concern themselves with documenting whether staff members deliver care; however, they should also be concerned with *how* they deliver it. It is important to note that we are not advocating the intentional display of fake employee affection, sociologically known as "emotional labor" (Hochschild 1983). We are merely advocating that interactions take on less of a bureaucratic tone and carry more of a human one. *Orient employees to bureaucracy.* Everyone involved with nursing homes should gain an understanding of how bureaucracy influences their organization. Administrators and other staff should become aware of ideas associated with bureaucratic rituals. They should gain an understanding, through training, of how bureaucratic rituals facilitate resident neglect and abuse. Employees in nursing homes may engage in maltreatment generated by rituals of bureaucracy without even knowing why.

We also suspect that many staff members experience high levels of stress in their jobs as the result of bureaucratic rules and procedures without realizing that such conditions create work pressure. Executive directors could, through periodic training sessions, orient staff to bureaucratic concepts and the potential problems created by bureaucratic organizations. Then the director or some other staff member could carry out a needs assessment to identify bureaucratic problems and ritualized behaviors that employees could reduce within state and federal guidelines.

Involve staff in organizational change. Once staff members are oriented to bureaucracy, encourage workers at all levels to continually reflect on and assess how work conditions can lead to detrimental outcomes. Involve employees in a collective effort to rethink how bureaucratic organizations operate and how they can be changed to enhance the lives of residents. Facilities could do this through informal discussions with administrators and supervisors, meetings, or suggestion boxes. If suggestions are made by staff members, then upper-level staff should take the suggestions seriously. In some cases, the staff actually caring for residents on a daily basis may have the best and most accurate insights into the small, daily ritualized practices that affect people in nursing homes in both constructive and harmful ways.

Orient residents and family members to bureaucracy. Residents and loved ones should also be oriented to bureaucracy. Administrators should make a point of discussing, in simple terms, the bureaucratic dynamics of their facilities. This includes basic organizational ideas and specific information about the facility. When facilities admit a new resident, a pamphlet with a flowchart detailing who does what in the home and a summary of facility-specific rules would be beneficial for residents, family members, and any other potential visitors. The goal should be to give residents and family members a better idea of how the facility operates, but also provide them with an increased understanding of how organizational dynamics can inadvertently lead to care-giving problems. We are aware of many situations where family members complain about visiting hours, meal times, or what items can be brought to family members. They don't realize they are complaining to the wrong person or that the rules they are violating went unnoticed in the paperwork they filled out during the complex admittance process.

Assign a facility greeter. Our research indicates that having someone greet people as they enter nursing homes would be beneficial. The greeter could be a volunteer resident and could wear a vest or other garment to denote his or her official status. Greeters would be able to meet with and direct family members and other guests who walk in the door, and could act as a liaison between visitors and staff when minor problems or questions concerning bureaucratic issues arise. Greeters could also help visitors with organizational questions by providing additional copies of the flowchart that details the duties of nursing home staff. Finally, they could help identify key personnel, such as the head nurse, the section nurse, or the on-duty supervisor, if a visitor has special questions or concerns about the resident they are visiting.

Revise staff policy, wages, and rewards. Hire more CNAs. Research indicates that organizations cannot achieve true "culture change" if they do not hire enough employees to adequately implement it (Lopez 2006b). Pay lower level employees more. This would help decrease turnover problems. Reports indicate that turnover among CNAs reaches rates as high as 97 percent (Deutschman 2005). Higher pay might also decrease the economic pressures that lower level staff feel. Such pressures can lead them to supplement their resources through criminal rituals such as property theft from residents. Also, provide merit pay when staff members perform in a way that discourages physical neglect. Moreover, provide them with extra funds if they act to encourage emotional support. In other words, provide them with incentives to meet the socio-emotional needs of residents. Money needn't be the only incentive. Facilities could utilize symbolic honors and formal recognition of employees who go against the bureaucratic tide and treat residents in especially humane and caring ways. Introducing positive sanctions would encourage RSPs that improve the quality of life of residents.

Reduce specific job/task mentality among staff. As our study shows, staff separation sometimes leads to employees neglecting the needs of residents when helping does not fit their job duties (e.g., administering medications or cleaning rooms). Administrators should emphasize to all staff that if a resident is in need with a minor problem (e.g., needing help to obtain a cup of ice cream or a glass of juice) any employee should help regardless of position in the organizational pecking order. Moreover, if a worker does not have the correct training to help with a serious issue, he or she should find someone who does. We believe that such efforts would promote more personalized ritualized behaviors, thus enhancing the well-being of residents. Highly ranked RSPs that focus on the personal needs of residents have the potential to change the thoughts and behavior of all staff members.

Increase upper-level staff and resident interaction. Studies indicate that for nursing homes to obtain positive resident outcomes, administrators need to embrace concepts promoting quality care (Ranz et al., 2004). Therefore, to reduce objectification, facilities should create measures for top staff to communicate with residents. Make it a requirement that they spend time during the workday visiting with residents. Doing so will counter the promotion of objectification and create an alternative ritualized logic in the facility, with the result that residents will feel that much more important and appreciated. Such practices would also create a model for other staff. In other words, administrators should facilitate in various ways ritualized behaviors that increase social communication and engagement between upper-level and lower-level staff and residents. They need to, as the colloquial saying goes, walk the walk and not just talk the talk.

Implement touch rituals. Human touch has the ability to increase the production of endorphins, which act as an anti-pain agent and reduce negative psychological symptoms related to stress. On this premise, many hospitals have incorporated formal massage therapy programs into health recovery plans (Anderson and Cutshall 2007). We recommend that nursing homes follow suit. However, we do not believe the utilization of touch should be limited to formal programs. It is possible to encourage employees, such as aides and nurses, to touch residents as much as possible in non-medical ways. The senior author recently visited his aunt in the hospital. She was suffering the effects of Crohn's disease. When he left her room, he gave her a light kiss on the forehead. She later sent him a note implying that the display of affection did a great deal to lift her spirits. We are not encouraging employees to kiss residents. Facilities need to consider touch rituals within today's legal context. We also want to note that we are not encouraging daily "hug-it-out" rituals to lessen the tension between staff and residents. What we are advocating is merely a higher level of friendly touches on the shoulder or back within legal reason to counter the poking and prodding characterized by medical-bureaucratic-based care.

Implement humor rituals. As *Reader's Digest* suggests, laughter is the best medicine. This idea is quite valid. Laughter has the same endorphin-producing capabilities just discussed, and scholars are advocating greater use of laughter in nurse–patient relationships. Greenberg (2003) argues that nurses can use humor, when appropriate, to produce laughter in health care environments. It not only has healing potential but also relaxes nurses when performing strenuous tasks and distracts patients during stressful procedures. Perhaps most important, shared laughter builds emotional support between caregivers and patients.

Be responsive to critically ill residents. When residents are sick or critically ill, and presumably dying, staff should check on them frequently. In other words, such residents should not be unattended for hours at a time. Even if a person is critically ill and there is no hope for recovery, employees should frequently check on the person in order to prevent discomfort or acute pain. The need to provide the highest quality of life possible should be a fundamental requirement, regardless of the condition or prognosis of the resident.

Acknowledge spirituality and death. Nursing homes should not overlook the importance of spirituality. Efforts could range from making religious services available to residents on a regular basis (e.g., having a weekly Sunday service), providing different kinds of reading materials to residents (e.g., books, audio books, or magazines dealing with spiritual matters), to recognizing staff who respond to residents' spiritual needs. Of course ensuring that religious figures such as ministers, rabbis, or priests regularly see residents who wish it is essential.

Facilities should also pay close attention to the way they deal with death. We are familiar with a situation where staff showed family members a potential resident a room that had a recently deceased person still lying in a bed. Some facilities will wheel deceased residents out through public areas, such as recreation or dining rooms, to ambulances. Some administrators make sure the first thing they ask family members of potential residents is what their funeral home preference is (see Hale 2005). Moreover, staff should acknowledge the death of residents. They should have work rituals that support the grieving process to let residents know their lives are important even though they live in institutions. For example, memorial services or at least death announcements would provide symbolic closure to the loss of someone in the organization. In addition, remember that anyone who was close to the deceased might need special counseling services, time off to grieve (for staff), or special accommodations during the grieving process (for residents with close bonds to the deceased).

Embrace resident narratives. Nursing homes should strive to record the stories of residents who are willing to share life histories. Such information could provide the basis for a personal narrative section in their charts. Some nursing homes already use personal narratives to help residents with dementia who are struggling to maintain a sense of identity (Moos and Bjorn 2006). However, the use of personal narratives does not have to be limited to residents with dementia. Facilities could have a picture of residents in an earlier stage of life to reinforce the idea they are working with people who experienced a rich life and are not just overly objectified elders. Residents who are able could also write their own biographies, which facilities could make available to both residents and staff. These narratives might illuminate individual residents' quirks and idiosyncrasies so that employees could better relate to them (for more, see Perkinson 2003 and Vesperi 2003). Publishing biographies in an organizational newsletter or simply distributing them among residents and staff or posting them in a common location would allow everyone access to people's stories.

Furthermore, facilities could contact a local newspaper and contribute to a column discussing the life of one or more residents on a weekly or monthly basis. This would mitigate the tendency to view residents as objects of work, while familiarizing the community with people in their institutions—factors operating against abuse and neglect. Along with making residents feel important and more autonomous, this would also make them feel more like a part of the wider community in addition to the nursing home itself. Again, the implementation of ritualized activities such as these, which occur quite often and are quite prominent (i.e., salient), would result in highly ranked rituals that affect both residents and staff.

Consider publishing newsletters. Nursing homes should create a newsletter to highlight important information about the facility and the people who work and reside in it. For instance, the newsletter could profile selected staff members and residents (including biographies of residents); identify upcoming special events; detail activities that will occur in the coming weeks in the nursing home; list the various supervisors, directors, and administrators in the facility; and discuss any important topical issues. Someone could write a monthly or quarterly newsletter and distribute it to all residents and staff within the home. The facility could even ensure a copy gets to family members and any others outside the facility who have a special relationship to residents.

While certain staff members would be ultimately responsible for the development of the newsletter, some residents could also be very involved in its production through, for instance, suggestions of topics, developing their profiles or biographies, writing about various topics, and identifying any persons they know outside the facility who would like to receive the newsletter. This would help increase the feeling among residents that they are useful, respected, and of value to the nursing home and others.

Promote empathy. Help staff members understand the lives of residents. This will build a sense of empathy and promote quality relationships. As mentioned, documentation concerning residents should include life histories. The organization should emphasize personal information just as much as information on medical conditions. In other words, staff members should realize getting to know residents involves more than just reviewing notes on their physical condition presented in a chart.

In addition, it might be of value to have all staff members, as part of their training, go through simulation exercises. As Deutschman (2005) argues, watching a training video is a passive exercise. As an alternative, aides and other workers could spend several hours in a mock resident room. We might even require facilities to have all staff, even administrators, tied down to the bed or wheelchair, fed meals, dressed in unappealing or inappropriate clothing, and ignored. This would literally give staff some idea of what it feels like to be dependent on others while sensitizing them to the fact that they are in their daily work rituals dealing with real people and not just objects. It might not be a bad idea to see if family members would participate in simulation rituals as well.

Counter isolation and loneliness from the inside. Take steps to ensure that employees do not leave residents alone in their rooms for hours on end. Facilities could develop systems to guarantee that residents receive a visit at least once a day (ideally several times a day if the resident wants) from a staff member, even if for only a relatively short period of time, in which some meaningful conversation takes place. This measure would help move the facility from a warehousing mentality to a more person-oriented mentality, where the personal and social needs of residents play a key role.

Counter isolation and loneliness from the outside. Engage as many outsiders in volunteer programs as possible. See if local high schools or colleges would send students to spend time with residents.

Moreover, encourage joint projects that build intergenerational ties. Consider oral history projects. Students could interview nursing home residents and write reports on their life histories. They could then edit the reports and donate them to local libraries for documentation purposes (see Ulsperger, Ulsperger, and Smith 2009). Nursing homes could start daycare centers to provide employees with reasonably priced child supervision. Able residents could volunteer to help take care of the kids. In addition, you could start an "adopt-a-grandparent program" to match up willing residents to willing children in hopes that they would interact in a quality way. You could also encourage resident involvement in as many community activities as possible. For example, if communities are commemorating people gone to war by placing ribbons on the trees in their yards, allow residents with loved ones at war to put ribbons up on trees located on the facility's grounds.

Counter loneliness and isolation with technology. Technology can certainly have both positive and negative sides. Regardless, it might be possible to carry out workshops in nursing homes designed to bring residents up-to-date with current technological trends. The cost for carrying out workshops would be minimal if students from local schools or colleges could hold them in order to gain experience. Building residents' familiarity with new technological tools of communication has the potential to bring them closer to others. For example, nursing homes could eventually build computer rooms and encourage residents to communicate with family members and friends via the Internet. This would involve hurdles such as reducing resident anxiety and unfamiliarity with new technology; however, it has some interesting possibilities. Imagine if capable elderly residents isolated in nursing homes had widespread ability to communicate with grandchildren through e-mail, Facebook, or MySpace. Moreover, would it not be interesting to see nursing home residents who are comfortable with technology having their own social networking sites with names like Graybook or Elder-Space? Aside from bridging communication gaps, recent research shows that Internet use improves the brain functioning of elderly people after just a few days (Gardner 2009).

Instilling modern technological skills into a resident's everyday rituals might also provide a higher level of openness and insight into the everyday workings of nursing home life. For example, though nursing home owners and employees might not like it, we would like to see residents with blogs detailing their daily care for the world to read about on the World Wide Web or a website for Internet-savvy residents to use in evaluating the facilities in which they live. College students have sites like ratemyprofessor .com, much to the chagrin of faculty members. Why should residents not be able to voice their opinions on similar websites? Ratemynursinghome.com has a nice ring to it.

Create consistency in ritualized social interaction. Our research indicates that facilities often rotate the areas where employees work. For example, one day a nurse's aide might work a particular wing of a nursing home and the following day work in an area on the opposite side of the facility. This process, sometimes known as "floating," can be good for employees who need flexibility in their jobs, but to the resident it reduces familiarity with employees and the associated work routines that they perform. It also bewilders residents who might, because of dementia, already be struggling with the confusion and strangeness of nursing home life. For these reasons, facilities should attempt to maintain consistent work areas for employees. Lessening exposure to inconsistent ritualized inter-action has the potential to create stability and cognitive consistency for residents. Of course, it would also provide the opportunity for more personal, intimate relations to develop between residents and staff. Family should also be aware that visit dynamics can create undue stress for residents. Gass (2004) implies that family should visit at regular intervals or not at all. When family members come sporadically, or during mealtimes or activities, it creates anomie in a resident's everyday schedule.

Reorganize the focus on rules to support autonomy. Because of errors and injuries in nursing homes, lawmakers have written a variety of nursing home regulations. Given the size and complexity of many facilities, rules provide the only mechanism for monitoring the quality of care. We certainly do not recommend that a facility should break the law and avoid rules. However, it is feasible and proper to call on administrators to acknowledge the negative impact of focusing too much on rules. We believe that the nursing home industry should work with policy makers and other concerned citizens to either reduce or revise nursing home rules. Research demonstrates that when nursing homes have productive, committed staff, an overemphasis on regulatory requirements and regulations can still undermine good care (Schnelle 2004).

Sometimes it may be beneficial to accept health risks in order to promote quality of life among residents. This could involve employees emphasizing residents' autonomy and the emotional, rather than the regulatory, side of care. Eliminate or reduce rules that restrict individuals from performing tasks for themselves. As just stated, this might involve accepting certain health risks for the benefit of quality of life. Be that as it may, let certain residents (who are capable) bathe themselves or (if not capable) receive person-centered baths. Person-centered baths focus on letting residents do as much as they can on their own, and then getting gentle, verbally supportive help from staff with bathing. Research shows that when organizations use person-centered bathing those involved in the bathing process view it as less of a burden (Hoeffer et al. 2006). Along with bathing, nursing homes could allow residents to periodically choose their own food, or part of a meal, such as their dessert or the main course. Along with the CNAs who provide most of their hands-on care, always allow residents to go to their own "plan of care" meetings so they have input into how their lives are organized. Let them help with various tasks in the nursing home. This will help them feel like they are caring for others as well as making a genuine contribution to the facility, even as they themselves are being cared for. In addition, let them, when feasible, have access to their own charts. Rigid and strictly enforced rules that promote dependency for medical reasons should not be the focus. Instead, facilities should try to, within reason given the needs and conditions of individuals, promote RSPs that stress autonomy and emotional needs.

Another aspect of supporting autonomy should include the understanding that not all residents want to participate in social activities offered by the facility. Stated quite simply, not everyone is the same! Gerontology's activity theory suggests that successful aging occurs when older adults remain socially engaged. However, we find that some residents are happier when they can develop their own personal rituals of behavior and not have employees force them into patterns of interaction promoted by the facility. Moreover, gerontology's continuity theory implies that people have a healthier aging process when they can continue activities they have been familiar with throughout the course of their lives. For example, residents should be able to decide if they do not want to participate in bingo or attend religious services. If they want to stay in their rooms and read or paint because that is what they did for pleasure before entering the nursing home, then they should be encouraged to do so. Forcing all residents to participate in structured activities takes away personal choice and identity, furthering bureaucratic objectification.

Allow residents to have official duties. Building upon the previous point we would argue that residents would greatly benefit from being allowed (and encouraged) to assist with various formal duties in the nursing home. By being involved in and contributing to the "official" functioning of the facility, individuals would personally benefit from the knowledge that they have made a substantial contribution to the needs of the organization and the care of others. Of course, they should also be periodically recognized and thanked for their contributions with announcements at dinner, in special meetings for everyone in the nursing home, or in newsletters.

Residents have the ability to engage in various duties. As already suggested some could serve as greeters to provide useful information to visitors. Another duty could involve helping to monitor the outdoor area, or assisting anyone who needs it. This might include helping the incapacitated through the doorway, calling for staff assistance if someone should fall while outside, and providing company to those who are lonely. Some residents, in a formal role, might also be able to assist the social director in developing recreational activities or in organizing and carrying them out. They could have positions where their responsibility involved helping to hand out supplies, helping to choose a particular video to show on a large screen television by soliciting suggestions from other residents, playing the video at a scheduled time, or organizing card games. Residents might also help distribute and collect reading materials from those who cannot leave their rooms.

Allow residents input into their program of care. Another point deserving further elaboration involves the desirability of having residents provide official input into their program of care and the kind of activities they want to engage in at the nursing home. Facilities could do this easily in various ways. A formal meeting with an administrator or head nurse upon entry is one option. Informal meetings with various staff persons at the time of entry or after the resident settles in is another. We believe these discussions should occur periodically, and not just upon entry to the home.

Participants could broach various issues, ranging from general tastes and preferences to more specific interests or concerns. For instance, residents could provide information on whether they want to exercise in some particular way or go for walks either in or outside the facility; for example, walking around the block or at a nearby park with a staff member or a volunteer. Residents might provide information on whether they would like to go outside in a special outdoor area (discussed later in this chapter with architectural concerns) and whether they might need assistance doing so. They could also discuss activities and hobbies, whether they would like some type of assistance with anything from playing certain kinds of card games to raising and watering plants in their room, reading the newspaper, reading books, or listening to audio books. They could also share information about any special foods or snacks they really like.

The resident could also provide general information about themselves, their likes and dislikes, and the kind of person they are. Are they, for instance a very sociable individual or more private in nature? Do they like to participate in many social functions and/ or possibly religious group events or are they more comfortable being alone and engaging in more personal types of activities? Would they like individuals from a church such as a minister, rabbi, or priest to visit when they come to the nursing home? Are there special concerns they might have about life in the nursing home or are there special activities they would like to participate in as part of their program of care?

Utilize communication tools. Administrators and other staff should acknowledge the importance of devices like television and radios. Nursing homes do not typically provide televisions or radios to residents. Usually, it is the responsibility of family members to buy them (assuming there are family members available to assist the resident, which is oftentimes not the case). Facilities should provide at least a small set (i.e., television and/or radio) to any resident that wants one. This might include multiple sets if there are several residents in one room. A set of headphones for each resident would be necessary. This would not only benefit hearing-impaired residents, but also encourage independent decision-making through channel selection. As a result, residents will not have to stare at a television watching another person's program of choice or listen to that individual's favorite station. Nursing home residents also report that during certain hours the noise coming from employees and other residents is sometimes unbearable (Kidder 1993). Headphones for television viewing or radio listening could also provide a barrier for residents not interesting in hearing employees and roommates discuss medical problems or even serve as a shield to night screams from other, less-coherent residents during sleeping hours.

We should also note that having a set in each room would provide residents with open access to information concerning the community, country, and world at large. In recreation areas, wide screen televisions should also exist. The screen should be large enough for people with vision problems. The facility could show movies that residents request, not just ones donated by, for example, local daycare centers. It would even be possible to show certain movies and have group discussions about them afterwards. This would be intellectually stimulating and could promote a sense of community among residents.

Empower residents. Residents lack resources. They are cared for by others and possess few resources. One way to change this situation is to have residents provide input into employee evaluations at every level of the organization. This will create a greater degree of balance for staff-resident relations. It will motivate staff members to provide better care if residents can be involved in decisions such as whether a staff member deserves a raise, promotion, or special recognition for their job performance and relations with others. Such a change would contribute to ritualized activities among residents that increase feelings of autonomy while facilitating work practices among staff that focus on care and attention to those for whom they are responsible.

Introduce emotions into documentation. As our study clearly shows, documentation is one of the most important bureaucratic rituals in nursing homes. Of course, a facility cannot do away with documentation just as it cannot do away with rules, but emotional factors integrated into documentation might lessen the impact of objectification. For instance, facilities could still record facts concerning the delivery of care, but they also could document *how* they deliver it. Formally integrating "emotive notes" into charting procedures would enhance staff's awareness of residents' emotional health and help build up the bond between those working and those living in nursing homes.

The notes could involve brief commentary on the resident's emotional state. They could also include the feelings of the staff member toward the resident and any reflections on how those feelings influence job performance. Admittedly, this will probably take some extra time. However, the emphasis should not be on the quantity of note taking or work but on quality. In that spirit, facilities could also reward staff for developing personal relationships with residents and not for task efficiency. It might also be beneficial to encourage residents to keep a diary or simply some short notes on how they feel toward staff. If that is not feasible, then higher-level or other staff should periodically ask residents about their feelings and relations with different workers—how they treat them, whether they enjoy and benefit from interacting with them, or whether they are disappointed and frustrated by the way others relate to them. Ritualized practices such as these could enhance empathy between staff and residents and lower tension and misunderstandings between them. All of these efforts would foster more person-centered, emotionally sensitive RSPs in the daily activities of workers and residents.

Recognize that small things matter. Make an extra effort to attend to the small details making up the daily lives of residents. Perhaps the guiding principle for staff should be *"nothing is too small to consider."* Remember that these small concerns and events in the lives of people can have a powerful effect on their overall state of mind and comfort.

For instance, make drinks available during the day between meals, and instead of having a few choices such as water and juice available at a public dispenser in the dining room, expand the options to four, five, or six items. That way if someone wants, for instance, a cola, lemonade, coffee, water, or hot chocolate, he or she can likely get it. In this regard, having a coin-operated machine containing various sodas and juices is not sufficient. If residents are bed ridden, or incapable of moving their wheelchairs, then they must rely on others to go to the machine for them (which they may not do). Moreover, if residents are poor they may lack the economic resources to purchase a drink. Again, although this may appear to be a minor or trivial matter for the resident who really likes a particular kind of drink but lacks the wherewithal to obtain it, having such access can be a very important and gratifying experience.

Provide high-quality laundry service. Make sure laundry rooms and services do not lose people's clothes. Sometimes clothes are lost or misplaced and then simply replaced with whatever is available; that is, current or former residents' clothes. Moreover, sometimes employees improperly wash clothes, such as washing a wool sweater with very hot water, thus shrinking the item. All of these occurrences can undermine residents' sense of self-worth and control over things as basic as their ability to construct and shape their own personal appearance. For fully cognizant individuals, appearance is quite important, and the loss or inadequate cleaning of their clothing can be devastating. Another way of saying this is that the ritualized practice of dressing and managing one's appearance can be a very significant part of a person's daily life, and having that interfered with and undermined can be quite demoralizing.

Consider residents' desires when going to dinner. A major part of residents' lives in a nursing home involves the time spent eating three meals a day in a dining room area (aside from those instances where individuals' conditions require them to eat in their room). To get to the dining area, however, can be difficult because people often need assistance walking or moving around in a wheelchair. For this reason, staff must expend a relatively large amount of effort taking people to and from the dining room during the day. The process of moving people to this area for each meal normally begins before the meal is actually ready.

However, sometimes aides and other staff, for reasons such as the desire to accomplish this task in a quick, efficient manner, begin this process earlier than necessary. Employees sometimes move residents to the dining area half an hour or even up to an hour before a meal. This means that those individuals end up sitting at the dinner table for extended periods with nothing to do. Some people may like this. They may enjoy being in an open area for an extended time where can they observe the activities around them and perhaps talk to those seated next to them. Others, though, may not find this enjoyable. Some individuals may feel that sitting there is boring, uninteresting, and uncomfortable. Staff should recognize that some individuals do not enjoy this experience and would rather be in their own room on some occasions. A minor change in how soon employees take people to dinner would be good for residents because it would accommodate residents' personal desires.

Institute a system of accountability for hygiene. The hygiene of residents should be an obvious and vital necessity. It is basic to the well-being of people. Because many people in nursing homes have difficulty with personal cleaning and are incontinent, others must attend to their needs. This requires a great deal of time and energy. It is only natural given the demands placed upon staff that residents must wait before help arrives. Unfortunately, the waiting period is sometimes too long. Residents may go for hours, large parts of the day, and even all day, with some of their hygienic needs not adequately met. Based on our research, we believe that this probably happens more than people imagine. For instance, employees may not adequately clean a resident's teeth, if they are cleaned at all. Sometimes employees do not change adult briefs for long periods, or if an employee does change the brief, the employee might leave the person's soiled clothing and bed unattended to for hours. Besides being unhealthy and offensive, such a condition can increase a resident's sense of powerlessness and undermine their pride and feelings of independence and self-worth. This is why upper-level staff should institute a system of accountability and supervision to ensure that such practices do not occur. Someone needs to check throughout the day, on a systematic basis, to make sure employees meet the hygienic needs of residents.

Respond to the individual needs and tastes of residents. The bureaucratic nature of nursing homes, which emphasizes qualities such as efficiency, often means employees carry out procedures and practices in a uniform manner whether that involves everyone eating the same foods at the same time or getting out of bed at the same time in the morning. We believe that facilities should make every possible effort to accommodate the different, individual desires of residents. Even if this is challenging for organizations and some resist it, it is imperative that facilities address this aspect of institutional life as much as possible.

Such an approach is extremely important because it would recognize the unique, personal needs and desires of residents and would facilitate their engaging in personal and social behaviors that are meaningful and significant to them. Facilities can do this in a number of ways. Some of these have been previously mentioned in the discussion of other points (e.g., supporting autonomy) but given their importance, we re-emphasize them here. In line with green house trends, facilities could allow residents to choose some of the foods they eat, whether this involves individual meals or having input into the weekly or monthly schedule for the dinners that will be prepared. Facilities should allow residents who wish to smoke to do it, as long as they do it in areas that will not bother other people. Smoking could occur in outside areas and a special room in the facility with proper ventilation. If medical conditions allow, facilities should let select residents drink alcoholic beverages of their choosing. Of course, issues such as how much and when this occurs (for instance, an evening drink as opposed to someone inappropriately drinking throughout the day) would have to be addressed.

Some residents might also be able to decide when they get up and whether they want to eat breakfast, unless medical conditions dictate otherwise. Finally, nursing homes should provide a means to allow residents to pursue hobbies that are meaningful to them. What those hobbies might be could range from raising plants or flowers to collecting stamps, coins, or other items. Here, we feel it is also important to mention the importance of sexuality and intimate relationships.

As mentioned in Chapter 5, many employees and family members downplay the existence and importance of sexuality and intimacy among residents. From a sexuality perspective, employees need to be more respectful. Gass (2004) indicates employees routinely barge in on residents while they are trying to masturbate in private. He goes on to detail a situation in which an elderly man and woman who were formerly neighbors liked to cuddle, nothing more, for an hour or so every night before going to sleep. The nurses in the facility found the behavior offensive. The woman's family, dealing with the idea of their elderly mother acting intimately with someone other than their deceased father, demanded that employees keep the man away from her. Employees and family should do a better job of recognizing needs of sexuality and intimacy, especially since research shows elderly people with healthy intimate relationships have a more positive aging experience (McKenzie 2000). We think all of the above ideas relating to personal needs and tastes are feasible. Nursing homes just need to have the will to implement them. We think the result would be a richer and more fulfilling life for many residents.

Utilize anti-infantilization rituals. Many things already discussed have the ability to limit infantilization, such as the aforementioned points on care input and empowerment. We want to emphasize that facilities should start thinking about altering specific nursing home rituals that have the direct ability to reduce infantilization. For example, do not ritualistically speak to residents with a child-like tone. Some of them might appreciate it, but not all of them do. An aide told us a story about a former professor in a nursing home who had an elevated amount of frustration when staff used "baby talk" on him. When a television is on in a common area, have it playing something suitable for adults, not children, unless residents prefer to watch child-based programming. With activities that provide prizes for residents, make sure prizes are appropriate. Although some residents might have mental characteristics that make the possession of a baby doll or stuffed animal suitable, not all do. To increase individual resident decision-making dynamics, it might be important to ensure that residents always have multiple prize options for recreational games. Again, not all residents are the same.

Organize recreation around group goals. When possible, activities should promote common goals to increase the social cohesion among residents and staff. For example, an activity director could place a puzzle in a common area and residents, along with employees, could stop by in their free time and gradually work toward the puzzle's completion.

Make administrators aware of special responsibilities. Administrators and supervisors need to be aware of the special responsibilities they have in a nursing home. They should make efforts to solicit from residents, family members, and other guests their honest appraisal of the quality of care received by residents. People, including those who are more knowledgeable about the workings of health care facilities such as nursing homes, may be (somewhat ironically) reluctant to be critical or raise pointed criticisms about specific staff members. That is because they realize that residents are, some of the time, in a potentially vulnerable position and subject to abuse or neglect by workers angered by criticisms. This means that individuals in positions of authority must be constantly aware of the possibility of retribution, make continual and concerted efforts to communicate with residents and visitors to gain their trust and assure them of the need to be honest, and then deal effectively with problematic staff behavior. In other words, administrators should not assume that silence or lack of reports about abuse mean there are no problems of this kind occurring in the facility.

Administrators should take responsibility for residents who are alone. Administrators and supervisors should be equally aware of the fact that many times residents have no visitors, for any number of reasons. Such residents are completely alone and especially vulnerable. This places a special responsibility on administrators and other staff to safeguard the health of such residents. It also means that supervisors should cultivate an atmosphere where open lines of communication exist between them and lower-level staff so that concerned, conscientious staff feel encouraged to report to administrators any suspicions they might have about possible abuse or neglect of residents.

Integrate facility meetings. When certain meetings are short or topics they address are not of immediate importance, consolidate and streamline meetings and in-service training sessions. Do not schedule meetings and training sessions when resident care should be occurring. As documented in this study, the proliferation of meetings can have a number of negative consequences—detracting from interaction with and care for residents—for staff members, who often reluctantly must attend them.

Do not conduct "surprise" family meetings. Our research indicates that some facilities will spring unexpected meetings on family members when they are visiting loved ones. This technique may play to the advantage of the facility and its employees, but it leaves family members feeling ambushed and alienated, particularly in cases where the meetings involve problems related to the actions of family members.

Consider clothing design. To create a balance between appropriate dress and efficiency, it might be possible to design dignified and appealing clothing that is also conducive to the bureaucratic necessity of working quickly. This is an issue that warrants serious thought and attention, but as far as we know has been absent from discussions about policies, procedures, and practices in nursing homes.

Address the architecture. Often, nursing homes resemble hospitals because they are in an old hospital or builders constructed them with a bureaucratic or medical rationale in mind. Many have a central hub design with wings, akin to spider legs, sprouting off in multiple directions. Interestingly, this reflects the design of some of our nation's earliest prisons, such as Eastern State Penitentiary in Philadelphia (see DeLisi and Conis 2010). Regardless, nursing homes with these designs often resemble what sociologists refer to as "total institutions," social settings removed from public life that segregate residents from the outside world while regulating and controlling their behavior to extreme degrees.

The architecture and physical arrangements of such institutions can have various consequences. In a broader sense, we concur with those in the culture change movement who believe nursing homes should be smaller facilities so people have the ability to interact with fewer people and to do so with higher quality and greater likelihood of personalization characterizing everyday interaction. Moreover, poor architecture promotes bodily harm in a variety of ways. Small rooms inhibit the ability for residents to move around freely with a relatively low risk of injury. When rooms are small with multiple people living in them, the likelihood of harm is increased because in crowded areas residents are more likely to accidentally bump into furniture, doors, or other people. If more than a few people come to visit a resident, small rooms make interaction uncomfortable and overwhelming for residents and roommates alike.

While restructuring architecture in existing homes would be difficult, architecture should certainly be addressed in the construction of new facilities. Ideally, future federal funding would allow all residents the option of having their own large, private rooms. This would not only alleviate room-crowding issues but increase privacy as well. If federal guidelines prevent this, then facilities should at least have designated areas where residents and family members can feel safe having discussions in private without being bothered by other residents or staff. Regardless, we believe facility designers should concentrate like never before on how the physical layout of a facility negatively influences resident well-being and then consider the relevance of design and architectural arrangements on the ritualized behaviors of employees. Even in existing homes, some modifications could probably be made that would mitigate problems and improve the lives of residents.

Aside from room size, architectural modifications can involve both large and small changes, yet can be quite consequential. For example, feeding off the Eden Alternative idea, we believe that all nursing homes should have outdoor areas (enclosed and preferably expansive) that residents can conveniently visit whenever they wish. Ideally, such outdoor areas would have a yard with grass, trees, bushes, a smooth-surface walkway, chairs and benches, and perhaps other features such as a garden with water fountains or birdbaths. An example of a small change would be making sure that doorways throughout the facility have smooth floors, because individuals in wheelchairs cannot easily, if at all, go over irregular or raised floors in doorways. Without wheelchair-friendly doorways, residents in wheelchairs must again depend on staff, other patients, or visitors to help them navigate through such obstacles. Finally, centrally situating reading rooms, recreation rooms, phone rooms, and other important sections of the nursing home are highly desirable. Centrally locating such activity areas makes it easier for residents to engage in behaviors that may be quite significant to them—for example, reading or playing games or cards with others—and in fact may even encourage them to do so.

Institute mandatory reporting. Many states require psychiatrists, advocates, social workers, and other mental health professionals to report cases of maltreatment to Adult Protective Services (Daly et al. 2004). However, few nursing homes require in-house mandatory reporting. Our findings demonstrate that because hands-on care is not technically the job of certain nursing home employees, such as administrators or office workers, or it might not occur within the normal course of their duties, they sometimes ignore abuse that they hear of or observe.

This situation could be alleviated if facilities had an organizational requirement for all employees not already required to report (i.e., nursing aides, office managers, administrative assistants, custodians, maintenance workers, kitchen workers) to inform supervisors about any suspected abuse. Moreover, volunteer workers could be encouraged to do the same. The executive director of the nursing home could institute this requirement in a contractual form provided during the early stages of employment with the facility. Changes such as this one would cultivate an organizational culture where everyone expects others to seriously monitor and deal with abuse; that is, to engage in ritualized behaviors involving the detection and reporting of maltreatment.

Screen out uncaring employees. Consider the possibility of screening out people who do not have an emotive, caring logic when it comes to others. In other words, do a better job in considering personal character and do not just fill bureaucratic positions in the nursing home on the basis of only the managerial abilities of balancing checkbooks or turning a profit. Poxon (2004) notes that as an activity director, one of the worst administrators she worked under was a hardnosed ex-naval officer who made life miserable for employees and residents alike. For lack of a better phrase, he ran a tight ship, but the activity director did not think that was enough when working in a nursing home. We tend to agree. We are not advocating that good managerial skills are unimportant in nursing homes, but nursing homes should be places of personalized care, not focused on uncompromising logics that run contrary to that care. Moreover, the best scenario involves administrators and employees who have the same goals with respect to resident care. When administrators and other employees are not on the same page, facilities are more likely to experience high turnover rates. This is problematic, especially when considering that high administrator turnover rates tend to have a negative effect on the quality of care in nursing homes (Singh and Schwab 1998).

Screen out motivated offenders. Consider the possibility of doing a better job at screening out at-risk, unqualified employees. Some employees, such as untrained aides, have histories of physical violence. This fact, coupled with the bureaucratic facilitation of resident maltreatment, increases the possibility of nursing home neglect and abuse. If facilities can better pinpoint these potentially abusive individuals through enhanced background checks and individual evaluations, administrators could keep them from joining an organization where vulnerable, suitable targets of crime are readily available. If administrators decide to keep hiring at-risk, unqualified employees, we recommend they implement security measures that make residents harder to victimize. For example, they might consider putting security cameras in areas where aides frequently have time alone with residents to deter them from committing crimes. Keep in mind, administrators would have to balance this move with issues involving privacy.

Educate motivated offenders. Though not directly discussed in previous chapters, we think it is important to acknowledge how diversity issues might also contribute to neglect and abuse of residents in nursing homes. This includes employee–resident divisions based on intergenerational, racial, and gender themes. Tension between younger employees and older residents might be the result of differences based on generational values. Cultural misunderstandings may create an increased level of conflict between minority employees and, predominately white resident populations. Unspoken discomfort relating to employees providing intimate care to residents of the opposite sex might foster an embedded friction that strains the staff-resident relationship. Heterogeneous nursing homes must acknowledge this and provide cultural diversity workshops for employees and residents.

In terms of racial conflict, research shows that minorities have developed successful techniques to combat racial abuse by residents. Minority CNAs ritualistically neutralize resident racist attitudes by reframing them with a family-based logic. Viewing unruly residents as family members instead of objects of labor allows CNAs to provide quality care in the face of verbal assaults (Berdes and Eckert 2007). Employees need to be aware of, and discuss, successful techniques such as these, whether dealing with race, age, or gender conflict that leads to subsequent resident abuse.

Recognize the multiple types of offenders. Research indicates there are different kinds of offenders in nursing home abuse cases. Approximately 24 percent are "stressed-out" abusers. They, while experiencing the typical stress associated with resident care, are provoked by residents and retaliate with abuse. Around 28 percent are pathological tormentors. They tend to inflict emotional abuse on residents without provocation. The largest percent are serial abusers. They engage in the systematic sadistic abuse of residents. Making facilities aware of these different types of offenders will enable them to better scrutinize employee behavior with the obvious goal of weeding out serious, repeat offenders (see Payne and Gainey 2006).

Recognize the multiple origins of offending. We hope that we have gotten the idea across in other areas of this book that employees are not the only motivated offenders in terms of nursing home abuse. Residents also have the potential to harm employees, whether it is through sexual harassment or physical assault. In addition, resident-on-resident abuse also exists. In a recent case, a family sued a Chicago facility where a resident, a 21-year-old mentally ill convicted felon, raped a 69-year-old woman. The family argued the administrator tried to cover up the crime by saying the sex was consensual (Johnson 2009). Recently, states such as Virginia have drafted legislation aimed at better identifying sex offenders in nursing homes. Because approximately 700 convicted sex offenders live in America's nursing homes, the legislation requires nursing homes to provide official notice to employees and residents when a sex offender enters a facility (Rondeaux 2007). Regardless, another way to counter problems associated with this issue involves resident clustering. Here we advocate facilities better separate residents based on age, cognitive abilities, or criminal background. This will help employees know what to expect when dealing with residents of a certain competence level and lower the likelihood of, for example, younger mentally ill residents assaulting older, vulnerable residents.

Revive law enforcement initiatives. In the late 1970s, the U.S. Congress mandated the creation of state Medicaid Fraud Control Units (MFCU). The goal of MFCUs is to investigate questionable financial actions and maltreatment in nursing homes. State MFCUs typically operate through a state's office of the Attorney General. We believe they focus too much on the financial side of resident exploitation and not enough on abuse issues. The lack of focus on abuse issues results from judge disinterest in handling nursing home cases, state agencies not reporting suspected criminal abuse to law enforcement, and a lack of appropriate and consistent statutes tying nursing home abuse to criminal behavior (Hodge 1998).

Research shows that only a minority of states have consistent statutes on nursing home mistreatment. One study, which examined laws in 14 states and the District of Columbia, found all of the 27 dynamics of elder abuse existing in adult protective services literature (Daly and Jogerst 2006). We need more consistency in legal definitions of elder abuse. We should also train local law enforcement on investigative techniques involving nursing home maltreatment, especially physical abuse issues. Although some states require local coroners to investigate nursing home deaths with the assumption of criminal motive, we find that few actually do. More awareness from the criminal justice side of resident treatment is crucial.

Allow care at home if possible. One of the best alternatives to living in the bureaucratic culture of a nursing home is to reside in the familiar, personal, nonbureaucratic environment of one's own home. While this is what many people would prefer, the simple truth is that doing so is extremely difficult for reasons ranging from prohibitive economic costs to the practical and organizational challenges of finding enough competent individuals to provide around-the-clock care. Regardless, we believe that if the medical condition of an individual allows for it, she or he should have the choice to age at home. Home health care businesses currently exist in a variety of areas around the country. Limitations based on Medicare and Medicaid coverage requirements have hampered their growth. We, therefore, strongly urge people in general and especially those with personal or professional experiences involving the nursing home industry to advocate for government measures that would make home care for the elderly a more viable alternative.

We hasten to add that if such a development were to occur, this would not mean that nursing homes would disappear. A need for many facilities would still exist because some individuals' poor medical health (both physically and mentally due to conditions such as severe dementia, Alzheimer's disease, and so on) would require total supervision and the comprehensive care that could be most effectively provided by a nursing home. Some people may even still choose nursing homes over aging in place. For instance, someone who is alone yet desirous of contact with other people might find traditional nursing home care appealing. We caution that a bloated, bureaucratic home health system might develop problems similar to the ones discussed in this book regarding nursing homes. We should remember that an expansion of home services and support, whether provided by the nursing home industry or other organizations, should be subject to vigilance and a system of accountability to ensure that a ritualized bureaucratic mindset does not undermine the quality of that care.

Conclusion

We believe that in the first half of the twenty-first century one of the most important and urgent needs before us is to decrease, if not eliminate, the bureaucratic culture of nursing homes. We think our CARE model can contribute to the development of new ritualized behaviors that have the potential to, as other culture change provisions do, better promote the social, emotional, mental, physical, and spiritual health of nursing home residents. We believe the rituals in our model, along with others in the culture change movement, have the ability to help counter the dominance and influence of bureaucratic rituals that shape nursing home life and lead to maltreatment. We want to emphasize that many of our recommendations have a firm theoretical grounding since they involve the principles of structural ritualization theory—a sociological perspective we discussed in Chapter 2 that has a large and growing number of studies supporting it.

We recognize that some of our recommendations might be difficult to implement and perhaps seem unrealistic. However, we hope the value of our research lies not only in our suggestions to change nursing home culture, but also in the possibility that some of our recommendations will further stimulate a dialogue about the bureaucratic nature of nursing homes and its negative consequences. In that dialogue, we strongly urge concerned citizens, health care professionals, policy makers, scholars, and students to include the voices of the residents themselves. In many cases, their observations may be the most perceptive and relevant of all. We cannot emphasize enough that legislators, nursing home consultants, and citizens should give serious consideration now to the adverse influences of bureaucracy on elder care. Bureaucracy is aiding in the catastrophic treatment of nursing home residents. Resident care has been too bad for too long.

CHAPTER 9

THE BUREAUCRATIC BOOM

ARE THERE OTHER OPTIONS?

> Man is a creature who can get used to anything,
> and I believe that is the very best way of defining
> him.
>
> Fyodor Dostoevsky

Bureaucracy exists throughout American society, and for that matter, most societies in the world. Weber (1946) was right about the future of bureaucracy. We have experienced a bureaucratic boom. This book focuses on the relationship between bureaucracy and nursing home care, but we believe bureaucracy has its hands around the throats of many other organizational forms and is choking the life out of them. Unfortunately, as a society we insist on blaming individuals and fail to see the bureaucratic nature of certain events and social problems. The elder care catastrophe we discuss in this book is just a part of this trend. To further our point, we want to provide you with a few key examples illustrating the idea that America is going through a larger bureaucratic catastrophe. After presenting them, we conclude with a brief review of some literature relating to bureaucratic alternatives.

Bureaucratic Breakdown

In 1972, complaints surfaced that Ford Pintos were exploding upon rear-end impact. Evidence indicated that the people inside Pintos when they exploded experienced few, if any, impact-related injuries. However, many would end up burning to death when their car doors were crushed and inoperable. Reporters and attorneys in civil trials scrutinized top decision-makers at Ford, arguing that the "higher-ups" made a rational decision to continue producing the Pinto even though it had design flaws. Specifically, executives at Ford found that it would cost more than $100 million to redesign the Pinto but it would cost only an estimated $50 million in potential lawsuits if they chose to do nothing. They chose not to redesign (see Dowie 1977). On the surface, this appears to have little to do with bureaucracy. However, research performed several decades later revealed that there might not have been a specific series of cost–benefit analysis decisions leading to continued Pinto production. Employees in the Ford bureaucracy knew there was a risk in producing any vehicle. The Pinto was no different. Moreover, top-level employees were not the only ones to blame. By producing vehicles for years without any major problems, Ford normalized a bureaucratic logic of acceptable risk that touched every level, from design to production (Lee and Ermann 1999). So, was the Pinto fiasco the result of a handful of executive decisions or a circumstance built on bureaucratic dysfunction and unanticipated consequences?

In January of 1986, NASA launched the space shuttle Challenger. Just over a minute into its launch, it exploded. A part known as an O-ring failed to seal at liftoff in the right rocket booster. Everyone on board died, including a teacher selected for NASA's new Teachers in Space Project (Kent 1993). Research shows that problems with the O-ring existed as far back as the late 1970s. However, much like the Ford employees who developed a culture of acceptable risk, NASA administrators regularly let launches occur when O-ring issues were present. Workers normalized O-ring problems and did not act on them. Sometimes, as with the Challenger, employees would find O-ring problems and not share the information with employees in other departments, either because they themselves believed they were insignificant or because employees in other areas would question their credibility for bringing up what was believed to be a non-issue (Vaughan 1999). With the Challenger, this dysfunctional bureaucratic practice finally caught up with NASA. Did NASA want astronauts to die? Obviously not. However, did a bureaucratic dynamic contribute to astronaut deaths?

On September 11, 2001, millions of Americans were shocked when a group of terrorists hijacked multiple airplanes for use as tools of destruction. Two planes were on their way from Boston to Los Angeles. The hijackers managed to take control of the planes and fly them into the World Trade Center towers. With both planes crashing into the mammoth structures that defined the New York skyline for years, twenty crewmembers, more than one hundred passengers, a handful of terrorists, and thousands of Americans and foreign nationals in the buildings ended up dead. Terrorists flew another plane, initially leaving Dulles International Airport en route to Los Angeles, into the Pentagon, while a fourth, believed to be on its way to the White House, crashed in a rural Pennsylvania field. In total, the attacks resulted in nearly 3,000 deaths (Bernstein 2002). Research shows that before the September 11 attacks, the Federal Bureau of Investigation refused to share certain information related to terrorism with the Central Intelligence Agency. The National Security Agency did not want to share information freely with anyone. Moreover, bureaucratic figureheads suppressed credible warnings of pending attacks while putting information collection and citizen protection on the backburner. Instead, in true bureaucratic fashion, they chose to focus on the development of new technology, organizational growth, and budget expansion (Gertz 2002). So, did a national security bureaucracy designed to protect American citizens ultimately contribute to the worst attack to take place on American soil?

On December 2, 2001, Enron, one of the most powerful companies in the United States, filed for bankruptcy. The media framed Enron's corporate leaders, which included Ken Lay and CEO Jeff Skilling, as greedy executives who lied to investors and shifted company losses in order to create an image of profit making (Fusaro and Miller 2002). However, research reveals that the organizational culture of Enron at multiple levels promoted the normalization of questionable business and sexual rituals, an elevated sense of hubris, and the use of fictional movie imagery to neutralize negative feelings associated with illegal behavior. Lay and Skilling may have known unethical things were taking place within Enron. However, even traders on the floor lied to investors, did not feel like they would ever be caught committing fraud, and jokingly discussed their disreputable behavior as if it was just part of a fantasy world (Knottnerus et al. 2006). The top brass at Enron set the tone of behavior within the company. However, did bureaucratic rituals inundating the entire organization cloud employee judgment and ensure the company's implosion?

The Roman Catholic Church came under fire in 2002 when prosecutors brought criminal charges against Boston-area priests for sexually abusing underage boys. The position advocated by some Catholics is that only a small percentage of the clergy have been involved in the sexual abuse of minors. However, some analysts indicate that child sexual abuse is a widespread, systematic issue ingrained in the culture of the church. A few years after the 2002 media frenzy, more than 13,000 minors had accused some 5,000 priests of sexual misconduct (Lynch et al. 2004; Reese 2004). Do certain priests objectify church members like some nursing home employees do with residents? Does this objectification open the door to abuse? Is the church so complex that abuse can go unnoticed when it takes place at lower levels?

Hurricane Katrina struck New Orleans in the early morning of August 29, 2005. The city's levees, designed to keep floodwaters at bay, failed. Soon, a majority of New Orleans was under water and thousands of evacuations occurred. Estimates indicate the loss of life attributed to Katrina at around 2,000 (Dudley 2006). Analysts believe many of those lives did not have to be lost. They argue that before and after the storm, the government at local, state, and federal levels, in true bureaucratic fashion, let its own complexities and rules get in the way of proper evacuations and a swift, substantial response. Interestingly, while trying to make the hazardous area of New Orleans safer, the government increased its potential for the loss of life and property. Regardless, people continue to point the finger at then president, George W. Bush, even noting that the government's response to Katrina would have been different if the racial composition of New Orleans was different (Burby 2006; Cooper and Block 2007). During a nationally televised Hurricane Katrina relief benefit, the wildly popular rapper Kanye West even stated, "George Bush doesn't care about black people" (Pareles 2007). Not to downplay the obvious racial issues surrounding Katrina, but perhaps he should have stated, "*Bureaucracy* doesn't care about *any* people."

Seung-Hui Cho killed 32 people and wounded many others on the campus of Virginia Polytechnic Institute and State University in

Blackburg on April 16, 2007. He was one in a long line of people over the past decade to carry out a mass homicide in an educational context. When these events occur in a secondary school setting, as in the case of the Columbine High School massacre of 1999 in Littleton, CO, or in a university setting, many people like to explain the event with individual-based theories. Whether this reaction comes from society's denial of responsibility in producing killers or the pop-psych stream of self-oriented logic prevalent in contemporary times, the kneejerk reaction is that the only reason it happened is that there was something wrong with the murderer. However, as our other examples in the breakdown of the bureaucratic boom imply, organizational issues are just as relevant. Post-Virginia Tech research shows several people at the university knew Cho had problems. However, bureaucratic rules prevented them from speaking to criminal justice officials or employees in other departments due to the school's stringent rules on student confidentiality. Moreover, easy access to guns, violent media influences providing cultural scripts for killing, and cultural feelings of alienation for students produced in bureaucratic educational environments may be more relevant to school shootings like Cho's than many people realize (see Newman and Fox 2009; Roy 2009).

Weber (1946) bet big on bureaucracy years ago, and society, for better or worse, has dealt us a bureaucratic royal flush. Unfortunately, people can get used to anything, and we have gotten used to bureaucracy. It has turned into a taken-for-granted reality so much that we do not even question its growth, let alone how its dysfunctions lead to social ills. We choose to focus our finger pointing at a few corporate executives, a faulty machine part, a political figurehead, or a disturbed teenager. However, we should start questioning bureaucracy more intensely. We do not have to roll over for it. We can do a better job of asking the question: Are there any reasonable alternatives to bureaucracy?

Alternatives to Bureaucracy

While not intending to provide an exhaustive list, we want to identify a few ideas related to alternatives to bureaucracy. Weber actually originated some of the first. He argued that people would not be able to do much to curb bureaucratic growth or even do away with it; however, he did argue that the formation of certain groups geared toward recognizing and alleviating bureaucratic dysfunctions might help (Ritzer 2008b).

Weber believed intellectuals, scientists, business leaders, and the leaders of major bureaucratic organizations should make up bureaucratic task forces. These task forces, along with wise politicians, could speak out against, and develop programs in direct opposition to, the domination of bureaucracy (Sadri 1992). This leads us to believe government and its charismatic leaders offer hope in a bureaucratic age. We should be able to ask them if they can do anything about bureaucracy and they should respond, "Yes we can!" Notwithstanding Weber's faith in political opposition to bureaucracy, we are currently in an era where the political answer to bureaucratic ills seems to be more bureaucracy, not scaling back on it. Consider the bureaucratic dysfunction related to the September 11 attacks. The political solution was to create more bureaucracy—the Department of Homeland Security (DHS). DHS represents a restructuring of federal law enforcement, intelligence, and emergency response agencies. In all fairness, DHS has probably thwarted more terrorist activities than we will ever know. However, the one major event handled by DHS after September 11, Hurricane Katrina, does not give us too much faith in DHS as a new, more effective form of bureaucracy.

A more sweeping approach than using task forces or anti-bureaucratic politicians involves the total transformation of society. Such a change would involve a wide-reaching and radical change of many or all of the institutions of society. The most likely change here would involve the transition from a market-oriented, capitalist system to a socialist system. Incrementally, this may already be occurring. Convergence theory implies that as societies around the world progress, socialist ones become more capitalist, and capitalist ones become more socialist. In Europe, we see reflections of this shift in the development of the European Union (Nachtigal and Votavova 2002). In the United States, we currently see signs of it with the move toward a more socialized health care system. However, even Weber argued that socialist systems are not a viable option for alleviating the problems associated with bureaucracy. In fact, he argued that socialist-based systems create more red tape and extreme government oversight, which makes bureaucratic tragedies more likely (Ritzer 2008b). Consider the various countries throughout the world that have implemented socialist or quasi-socialist systems in the past 100 years (e.g., the Soviet Union, Eastern European communist countries, and China). One could argue they are more bureaucratic than the United States. Moreover, you could argue that bureaucratic, government organizations in these socialist systems lead to an exaggerated level of human objectification and a variety of problems associated with human rights violations.

Regardless of the preceding points, research indicates that even within a capitalist social system, bureaucratic alternatives can be viable. Consider grassroots worker cooperatives, corporate worker participation programs, and employee ownership plans. With worker cooperatives, workers invest in a business and democratically decide what is in the best interest of the business. Estimates indicate that 300 cooperative-based workplaces currently operate in the United States and they generate over $400 million in revenue each year. A key anti-bureaucratic theme with such cooperatives is that they are small businesses with employees who have high levels of cohesion while uniformly promoting organizational goals (U.S. Federation of Worker Cooperatives 2009). Large organizations house worker participation programs. With these programs, administrative leaders encourage employees at all levels to participate in decision-making. This includes the use of problem-solving groups with members from multiple areas of the organization who make policy recommendations to those at the top levels of the bureaucratic hierarchy. Employee participation programs orient themselves around just about any organizational issue, even the reduction of mental health problems associated with employment (see Kobayashi et al. 2008). Employee ownership plans encourage the use of employee stock ownership to, among other things, heighten loyalty and maximize worker production. Here, the idea is that if you own a part of the organization you work for, you are going to do a better job working for it. The trend started in the 1980s, and by the 1990s, around 6 percent of companies had employee ownership plans in place (Cramton, Mehran, and Tracy 2008).

Research shows that these alternative forms of economic workplace structure do have advantages. They increase job satisfaction and in some cases decrease turnover rates. However, they lose their effectiveness when used in larger organizational environments. They also create higher levels of absenteeism. When workers feel like they own a part of the company, they feel like they have a right to skip work when they feel like it. Workers also report missing more work because the strain of the personal responsibility they feel decreases their psychological well-being (Rothschild and Russell 1986).

From a more practical, organizational level, limited literature exists on specific bureaucratic reduction policies. One exception is Ken Johnston's work *Busting Bureaucracy* (1993). As a former IBM employee, Johnston used sociological and business-centered foundations to develop ideas on the limitation of bureaucratic problems in organizations. In his book, he argues that organizations should recognize bureaucracy is a problem, and then they should start using organizational models built on quality interaction. This includes goals related to flattening hierarchical structure by empowering organizational members at all levels, using guidelines for behavior and not stringent rules, and requiring individual departments to nest their individual missions within the larger organizational mission to streamline organizational ideologies. In addition, if top-level employees do not want to recognize bureaucratic problems or are not contributing to the betterment of the organization, replacing them might be necessary to change the tone of the organization.

A new approach to bureaucratic alternatives originates from Bernard Phillips's work. Phillips, using the seminal ideas of C. Wright Mills (1959), helped to develop a new methodology in sociological analysis known as the Web/Part Whole approach. With it, the analysis of human action calls for a broad scientific analysis that, among other things, stresses the need for abstract concepts to explain these complicated social behaviors and processes, different kinds of empirical methods (i.e., qualitative to quantitative) to study and support those ideas, and using this knowledge to solve major social problems in modern society (proposals we completely agree with and are committed to). Building off this idea, and others presented in the *Advancing the Sociological Imagination* series with Paradigm Publishers (Phillips 2001, 2007, 2009; Phillips and Johnston 2007; Phillips, Kincaid, and Scheff 2002; Knottnerus and Phillips 2009), Phillips's view of bureaucratic alternatives focuses on the total transformation of individual worldviews.

Bureaucracy permeates our everyday lives so much, even when we are not around it; it shapes the ways we talk, think, and act, often for the worse. As such, Phillips explains we should replace bureaucratic worldviews that push us in the direction of limited, specialized communication and hierarchical relations with an evolutionary worldview characterized by deep, meaningful, expressive interaction patterns. Once a multitude of individuals stop thinking bureaucratically, bureaucracy will loosen its grip from the ground up, which has the potential to result in large-scale social change. Only then will we have the ability to truly control our lives and save society (for more, see Phillips and Christner 2009). This idea possesses a great deal of potential and could be critically important for society and especially individuals. Of course, getting large numbers of people to recognize their taken-for-granted bureaucratic thought and action patterns and then having them actively try to change them would require commitment, time, and a lot of effort.

The CARE model presented in the previous chapter also provides ideas that could serve as bureaucratic alternatives in areas other than nursing home care. We believe dysfunctional aspects of bureaucracy in nursing homes reflect the same kinds of bureaucratic dysfunctions existing in other organizations, whether they involve, for instance, rules and regulations influencing work rituals, hierarchical duty specialization, documentation-driven communication patterns, or themes of human objectification. Therefore, our recommendations, which are oriented toward an emphasis on the emotional component of interaction, hiring practices based on anti-bureaucratic ideologies, cultural diversity training, and employee rewards for nonbureaucratic behavior could promote humane-based behavior in other social settings.

We realize that all organizations are not the same; however, the core themes related to alternative RSPs in the CARE model can have applications in other bureaucratic settings like hospitals, government agencies, mental health facilities, corporations, the criminal justice system, educational systems, sports teams, or even religious establishments. That is why it is important that our approach is focused yet flexible. The analytical framework (grounded in structural ritualization theory) with its emphasis on rituals can be applied to various bureaucratic systems operating in different organizations, the specific kinds of bureaucratic RSPs occurring in them, and the goal of enacting alternative ritualized activities.

What this would entail is an analysis of the dominant bureaucratic rituals operating in an organization and the effects they have on people, particularly the negative consequences of these RSPs and the ways they impede the workings of the organization. Attention then should be given to what kinds of alternative goals and rituals are desired. Finally, one would need to determine the various ways these alternative ritualized practices could be cultivated.

All the important dimensions of the organization should be considered, including the organization's rules; formal arrangements (e.g., authority system, types of positions and their overall structure); duties of workers; nature of documentation; key units, groups, and individuals involved in the transmission of rituals; training and hiring of personnel; reward system for employees; nature of the interaction occurring among all persons including individuals who may be serviced by and possibly reside in the organization; situational dynamics and pressures; physical layout; wider social environment affecting the bureaucracy; and so on. These different aspects of the organization can play a crucial role in both facilitating bureaucratic rituals and alternative non-bureaucratic rituals.

By addressing these issues in the manner just prescribed we believe it is possible to significantly alter the bureaucratic ethos and ritualized behaviors of people within many if not all organizations. The central role ritual plays in social behavior and organizational dynamics provides us with not just an analytical framework for better understanding bureaucracy and its problems but also a tool for changing in a pragmatic fashion the harmful and unproductive consequences of bureaucratic systems.

Conclusion

A great deal of pessimism about the effects of bureaucracy has developed over the past century. Recent events, such as the British Petroleum oil disaster in the United States, have certainly not elevated the public's confidence in bureaucratic responses. However, we do not have to have a gloomy view of what will surely be an organization-dominated future. We are optimistic about the potential to lessen the negative effects of bureaucracy, or better yet alter the course of the ongoing bureaucratic boom. The bottom line, from our perspective, is that if humans can create bureaucratic structures, we can also change them with ritualized alternatives to bureaucracy.

This may appear to be a difficult task, but we do not believe it is an insurmountable challenge. What is essential is that we start elevating our commitment to recognizing bureaucracy and confronting its unanticipated consequences before inevitable future bureaucratic breakdowns occur. If we do not, countless more people will suffer the catastrophic consequences of bureaucracy, not just in nursing homes, but also in a multitude of other areas driven by bureaucratic dynamics.

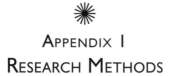

APPENDIX I
RESEARCH METHODS

The topic of nursing home abuse and neglect is tough for researchers to tackle. Entering a nursing home and getting honest results would be difficult if you told the administrator you wanted to go around the facility and survey employees with "yes" or "no" questions on maltreatment. Therefore, we chose to study this topic by using low-profile methods. This included a content analysis, observation techniques, off-site employee interviews, and the distribution of open-ended questionnaires.

For our content analysis, we used Van de Poel-Knottnerus and Knottnerus's (1994) literary ethnography process. We initially developed our scope of literary sources by finding every piece of literature on everyday nursing home life we could using library and Internet search engines. This included books, book chapters, chapter sections, and articles written by academic researchers and non-academics that lived in, had family members in, or worked in nursing homes. With a core of sources from the past 40 years, we thoroughly examined the references of each source for additional references. With an intense search for all literature on nursing home life complete, we ended up with fifty-three sources appropriate for analysis. Then we separately and thoroughly reviewed portions of the literature while sitting in non-distracting environments to obtain a high level of concentration. Thanks to our past research on long-term care and personal experiences volunteering in and having family members in nursing homes, we were comfortable with much of the language and technical jargon in the sources. Next, we identified prominent themes. We initially found more than one hundred themes involving anything from general work practices, such as employee charting, to specific trends on issues, such as family involvement and privacy. At this point, we started to notice strong themes related to organizational processes and resident maltreatment. We took written notes on these themes and kept track of where key examples existed.

Focusing on organizational work and resident maltreatment themes, we read and reread all of our sources and coded examples of bureaucratic operations and resident maltreatment along the way. Before coding, we decided to use specific analytic constructs to develop concrete operational definitions. For organizational processes, we relied on Max Weber's (1946) formal definition of bureaucracy, which includes aspects of hierarchical relations, rules, documentation, and efficiency. For resident maltreatment, we relied on previously developed definitions of elder maltreatment that led to distinctions between emotional, physical, and verbal neglect and abuse (see, for example, Pillemer 1988). We coded paragraphs and larger grammatical units, such as paragraph sequences, and kept track of the number of times rituals of bureaucracy and maltreatment appeared and contained certain intense examples to use as descriptive illustrations for our findings. Finally, we sought contextual confirmation to get an idea of the trustworthiness of our research. Here, we reread portions of our literary sources one last time, checking to make sure that our final ideas on nursing home bureaucracy and maltreatment accurately reflected our sources. We also carried out discussions of our findings with other people having experience with nursing homes to see if our findings matched their perceptions.

With respect to observational data, the senior author interned with two executive directors for six months at a nursing home in the northeast corner of Arkansas from January until June of 1999. At the time, the facility had 113 beds and 94 residents and was part of one of the largest nursing home chains in the United States. Field notes from this experience focused on organizational dynamics and included the documentation of administrative interaction in offices and during meetings. At times, work involved task support for the executive director, social service director, activity director, and nursing staff. The senior author then served as a volunteer for the social service director in a 125-bed facility with 58 residents in the north central part of Oklahoma from August to December of 1999. Observations and accompanying field notes were restricted to interaction with residents and lower-level staff members such as aides. The second author's personal observations occurred while his mother was living in a nursing home in north-central Oklahoma. She was in a nursing home from April 2007 to August 2008.

Student researchers collected interview information from 2008 to 2009. They met with people who worked in or used to work in nursing homes. For those working in nursing homes, interviews took place off-site. In other words, we made sure they did not occur at the facilities where the interviewees worked. Ensuring interviewees complete anonymity, the student researchers asked workers questions geared toward the themes of bureaucracy and resident maltreatment we found in our content analysis. For our questionnaires, we were able to locate former nursing home employees and resident family members through informal discussions about our research with colleagues. In the summer of 2009, we contacted each person to see if he or she would be willing to participate in this research. If the person agreed, we ensured confidentiality and mailed the participant questions related to our research. We sent every person interviewed a questionnaire. They all signed a consent form with provisions approved by an institutional review board.

APPENDIX 2
A BRIEF GUIDE FOR
NURSING HOME SELECTION

This appendix details ten issues we feel are important when a family member is looking to turn to a nursing home for a loved one's elder care and things they should do after a loved one starts living in a facility. We recommend readers seek additional information on these issues and others from agencies such as the Centers for Medicare and Medicaid Services (http://www.cms.hhs.gov/), the National Association of Area Agencies on Aging (http://www.n4a .org/), and local Area Agency on Aging offices.

1. *Plan ahead.* If you think a loved one might have to enter a nursing home in the future, do not be deceptive about what is happening. Openly discuss the issue as soon as possible and discuss your loved one's facility of choice. Also, remember that nursing home care is expensive. As discussed in Chapter 3, within months of entering a nursing home, many residents spend all of their savings and have to apply for Medicaid. Speak with a financial advisor years ahead of time if possible in order to plan for the

financial impact of nursing home care in a way that will minimize unnecessary fiscal loss for the resident and close family members.

2. *Review government survey information.* Check the Nursing Home Compare system at www.medicare.gov/NHCompare or call 1-800-633-4227. You can obtain detailed survey information on the 150 regulatory standards measured in nursing homes that receive federal funding. This includes data on everything from fire safety to staff ratio infractions. You can also find out information such as ownership type, the number of beds in a facility, and the number of residents.

3. *Talk to friends and your local ombudsman.* We find that often people who find good nursing homes for loved ones do so by word of mouth. Speaking with friends who have loved ones in nursing homes will also let you know which facilities to avoid. Your local ombudsman will work for the Area Agency on Aging. It is the ombudsman's job to mediate conflicts between residents, families, and nursing homes. They will have a gauge of good and bad facilities in your area. However, be aware that some have better relationships with facility administrators than residents and families. That may skew opinions.

4. *Perform an on-site visit.* Go for an informal visit to the nursing homes you are considering. If possible, go more than once at different times during the day or week. In addition, take the potential resident with you if you can. Ask to speak with the director and key in on how they interact with staff. Also, note the director's demeanor in answering your questions. Find out if the director's focus is on resident care or bureaucratic and financial issues. In addition to speaking with the director, ask to speak with

other staff without the director present. Speak with the facility's social service director and find out what rules and regulations you will have to abide by as a resident's family member. Ask to speak with a few residents when you visit potential nursing homes. The key phrase here is "a few." Some facilities will direct you to someone they believe paints the best picture of the facility, so be sure and have some variety.

5. *Visit after admission.* Be sure and go see your loved one after admission at regular intervals. Aides interviewed for this research indicated that people who have regular visitors get better care. Moreover, the post-admission adjustment will be hard. Your loved one's sense of self will change, and we feel that the more continuity you provide them in terms of maintaining relationships the better. When you visit, have a dependable, regular schedule. Residents would sometimes rather not have visitors at all than be in a situation where they think someone is coming and then the person does not show up. Do not bring large numbers of people to visit. Nursing home rooms can be small, and large numbers of people cramming into them for visits can be overwhelming for a resident. Also, try to visit when residents are not preoccupied with activities such as eating or therapy.

6. *Heed to happiness.* We think you should strive to help maintain a family member's sense of self after they have entered a nursing home, but also recognize healthy changes in self-concept related to new interaction patterns. For example, residents sometimes find love after entering a nursing home and take on the status of boyfriend or girlfriend for the first time in years. Just because you are uncomfortable with your aged mother or father building

a romantic relationship with someone while living in a nursing home, you should not demean it if it provides your loved one with a positive aging experience.

7. *Educate staff.* Tell the nurses and aides what your loved one's likes and dislikes are. Whether it is a favorite cup to drink out of before bed or a nickname they do not like, many employees do not know what a resident's quirks are and residents sometimes feel uncomfortable revealing them. If your loved one is okay with it, we also encourage you to fight objectification by telling nurses and aides about your loved one's life history.

8. *Be amicable.* Build positive relationships with staff. When talking to them, let them know you recognize the bureaucratic constraints they work under. If you have problems with an employee, handle the situation with the best attitude you can muster. Remember that your loved one will have to deal with the consequences of any bad situations you contribute to as soon as you walk out of the facility's doors. You are not there 24 hours a day, but the employees you rub the wrong way are.

9. *Do not deflect guilt.* Do not overcompensate for your feelings of guilt related to placing a loved one in a nursing home by picking apart every aspect of care provided by staff. Some instances of maltreatment, such as intentional abuse, need serious attention. However, after reading this book hopefully you understand that occasional, unintentional aspects of neglect are just part of nursing home culture. That does not make them acceptable; however, you should remember that good nurses and aides doing their best sometimes slip up as a result of everyday work pressures.

10. *Recognize excellence.* We want to emphasize again that there are wonderful nursing homes. If you have a loved one in one of these homes, show your appreciation. Give employees little notes, or perhaps suitable gifts, for providing good care. As mentioned in Chapter 8, we think that recognizing excellence in employee care has the ability to motivate employees to continue providing quality treatment. Fight the negative press given to nursing homes so frequently by writing a letter to the local newspaper pointing out the good care your loved one is receiving.

REFERENCES

AAHSA. 2008. "AAHSA History" (About the American Association of Homes and Services for the Aging). Washington, DC: AAHS. Retrieved July 1, 2008 (http://www.aahsa.org/about_aahsa/history/default.asp).

AHCA. 2008. "About Us" (Welcome to the Alliance for Quality Nursing Home Care site). Washington, DC: ACHA. Retrieved July 1, 2008 (http://www.aqnhc.org/contact.html).

Achenbaum, W. Andrew. 1978. *Old Age in a New Land: The American Experience Since 1790*. Baltimore: Johns Hopkins University Press.

Adams, Jim. 2000. "Nursing Home Nurse Accused of Raping Comatose Patient." *Star Tribune Newspaper of the Twin Cities,* April 21, p. 5B.

Allison, Christopher. 2007. "Bureaucratic Personality." In *The Blackwell Encyclopedia of Sociology,* ed. George Ritzer, 378–380. Malden, MA: Blackwell.

Amirkhanyan, Anna, Hyun Joon Kim, and Kristina Lambright. 2008. "Does the Public Sector Outperform the Nonprofit and For-profit Sectors? Evidence from a National Panel Study on Nursing Home Quality and Access." *Journal of Policy Analysis and Management* 27(2): 326–353.

Amon, Mike and Tom Zambito. 2001. "Nursing Home Deaths Soar." *New York Daily News,* February 15, p. 31.

Anderson, Geoffrey, Sudeep Gill, Michael Hillmer, Paula Rochon, and Walter Wodchis. 2005. "Nursing Home Profit Status and Quality of Care: Is There Any Evidence of an Association." *Medical Care Research and Review* 62(2): 139–166.

Anderson, Patricia and Susanne Cutshall. 2007. "Massage Therapy: A Comfort Intervention for Cardiac Surgery." *Clinical Nurse Specialist* 21: 161–165.

Arnold, Thurman. 1935. *The Symbols of Government*. New Haven, CT: Yale University Press.

Barry, Theresa, Diane Brannon, and Vincent Mor. 2005. "Nurse Aide Empowerment Strategies and Staff Stability: Effects on Nursing Home Resident Outcomes." *Gerontologist* 45: 309–317.

Baxter, Cynthia. 2008. *Monkey See, Monkey Die*. New York: Bantam Books.

Bell, Catherine. 1992. *Ritual Theory, Ritual Practice*. New York: Oxford University Press.

Bellah, Robert N. 1968. "Civil Religion in America." In *Religion in America*, ed. William G. McLoughlin and Robert N. Bellah. Boston: Houghton Mifflin.

Bennett, Clifford. 1980. *Nursing Home Life: What It Is and What It Could Be*. New York: The Tiresias Press, Inc.

Berdes, Celia and John Eckert. 2007. "The Language of Caring: Nurse's Aides' Use of Family Metaphors Conveys Affective Care." *Gerontologist* 47: 340–349.

Bernard, Thomas J. 1992. *The Cycle of Juvenile Justice*. New York: Oxford University Press.

Bernstein, Richard. 2002. *Out of the Blue: The Story of September 11, 2001*. New York: Times Books.

Biderman, Albert D. and Albert J. Reiss. 1967. "On Exploring the 'Dark Figure' of Crime." *Annals of the American Academy of Political and Social Science* 374(1): 1–15.

Billups, Andrea. 2006. "Deadly Neglect: The Shocking Truth About What's Going on in America's Nursing Homes." *Reader's Digest*, December, pp. 97–103.

Blau, Peter and W. Richard Scott. 1963. *Formal Organizations: A Comparative Approach*. London: Routledge and Kegan Paul.

Bloch, Maurice. 1989. *Ritual, History and Power*. Oxford: Berg Publishers.

Bova, Ben and Christian Noble. 2007. *Immortality: How Science Is Extending Your Life Span and Changing the World*. Beverly Hills, CA: Phoenix Books.

Brawley, Elizabeth. 2007. "What Culture Change Is and Why an Aging Nation Cares." *Aging Today*, July–August, pp. 9–10.

Brawley, Elizabeth and Paul Kleyman. 2007. "Outcomes on Research Alternatives." *Aging Today*, July–August, p. 11.

Brody, Elaine. 1984. "Informal Support Systems in the Rehabilitation of the Handicapped Elderly." Paper presented at Aging and Rehabilitation, a national conference. National Institute of Handicapped Research, National Institute of Mental Health, National Institute of Aging, Washington, DC.

———. 1990. *Women in the Middle: Their Parent-Care Years.* New York: Springer.

Brooks, Charles H. and John A. Hoffman. 1978. "Type of Ownership and Medicaid Use of Nursing-Care Beds." *Journal of Community Health* 3: 236–244.

Brown, Martyn. 2007. "The Hospice Cat That Can Predict Who Will Die Next." *The Express,* July 27, 2007.

Bryman, Alan. 2005. "McDonaldization." In *Encyclopedia of Social Theory,* ed. George Ritzer, 485–486. Thousand Oaks, CA: Sage Publications.

Buhler-Wilkerson, Karen. 2003. *No Place Like Home: A History of Nursing and Home Care in the United States.* Baltimore, MD: Johns Hopkins Press.

Burby, Raymond. 2006. "Hurricane Katrina and the Paradoxes of Government Disaster Policy: Bringing About Wise Governmental Decisions for Hazardous Areas." *Annals of the American Academy of Political and Social Science* 604: 171–191.

Burling, Stacy. 2007. "Genesis Receives a Newer, Higher Bid." *The Philadelphia Inquirer,* April 26, p. C1.

Burns, Tom and George M. Stalker. 1961. *The Management of Innovation.* London: Tavistock.

Carlson, Eric and Katharine Bau Hsiao. 2006. *The Baby Boomer's Guide to Nursing Home Care.* Lanham, MD: Taylor Trade.

Cicirelli, Victor G. 1990. "Family Support in Relation to Health Problems of the Elderly." In *Family Relationships in Later Life,* ed. Timothy H. Brubaker, 212–228. Newbury Park, CA: Sage Publications.

Clark, Burton. 1972. "The Organizational Saga in Higher Education." *Administrative Science Quarterly* 17: 178–184.

Clegg, Stewart. 2007. "Bureaucracy and Public Sector Government." In *The Blackwell Encyclopedia of Sociology,* ed. George Ritzer, 376–378. Malden, MA: Blackwell.

CMS. 2008. "Special Focus Facility Initiative." Centers for Medicare and Medicaid Service, Washington, DC. Retrieved July 1, 2008 (http://www.cms.hhs.gov/CertificationandComplianc/Downloads/SFFList.pdf).

Cohen, A. 1993. *Masquerade Politics: Exploration in the Structure of Urban Cultural Movements.* Oxford: Berg Publishers.

Cole, Thomas R. 1987. "Class, Culture, and Coercion: A Historical Perspective on Long-term Care." *Generations.* Summer: 9–15.

Coleman, James William. 1985. *The Criminal Elite.* New York: St. Martin's Press.

Collins, Dave. 2009. "Waves of New Fund Cuts Imperil U.S. Nursing Homes." *Associated Press Release,* October 4.

Collins, Randall. 2004. *Interaction Ritual Chains.* Princeton, NJ: Princeton University Press.

Committee on Energy and Commerce. 2008. *In the Hands of Strangers: Are Nursing Home Safeguards Working?* Subcommittee on Oversight and Investigations, Washington, DC.

Conrad, Kendon, Patricia Hanrahan, and Susan L. Hughes. 1990. "Survey of Adult Day Care in the United States." *Research on Aging* 12: 36–56.

Cooper, Christopher and Robert Block. 2007. *Disaster: Hurricane Katrina and the Failure of Homeland Security.* New York: Times Books.

Cramton, Peter, Hamid Mehran, and Joseph Tracy. 2008. "ESOP Fables: The Impact of Employee Stock Ownership Plans on Labor Disputes." *Staff Reports—347,* Federal Reserve Bank of New York.

Daly, Jeanette and Gerald Jogerst. 2006. "Nursing Home Statutes: Mistreatment Definitions." *Journal of Elder Abuse and Neglect* 18(1): 19–39.

Daly, Jeanette, Gerald Jogerst, Margaret Brinig, and Jeffrey Dawson. 2004. "Mandatory Reporting: Relationship of APS Statute Language on State Reported Elder Abuse." *Journal of Elder Abuse and Neglect* 15(2): 1–21.

D'Aquili, Eugene and Andrew Newberg. 1999. *The Mystical Mind: Probing the Biology of Religious Experience.* Minneapolis, MN: Fortress Press.

DeLisi, Matt and Peter Conis. 2010. *American Corrections: Theory, Policy, and Practice.* Boston, MA: Jones and Bartlett.

DeSpelder, Lynne Ann and Albert Lee Strickland. 2009. *The Last Dance: Encountering Death and Dying.* Boston, MA: McGraw Hill.

Deutschman, Marian T. 2005. "An Ethnographic Study of Nursing Home Culture to Define Organizational Realities of Culture Change." *Journal of the Health and Human Services Administration* 28(2): 246–281.

Diamond, Timothy. 1992. *Making Gray Gold: Narratives of Nursing Home Care.* Chicago: University of Chicago Press.

Dolinsky, Elaine and Herbert Dolinsky. 2008. "Infantilization of Elderly Patients by Health Care Providers." *Special Care in Dentistry* 4(4): 150–153.

Donahue, Cecil. 2008. "Attack of the Consultants!" *Gentlemen's Quarterly*, September, pp. 288–290.

Dosa, David M. 2007. "A Day in the Life of Oscar the Cat." *New England Journal of Medicine* 357: 328–329.

Dowie, Mark. 1977. "Pinto Madness." *Mother Jones* 2: 18–32.

Dudley, William. 2006. *Hurricane Katrina*. Detroit: Greenhaven Press.

Duhigg, Charles. 2007. "At Many Homes, More Profit and Less Nursing." *New York Times*, September 23, p. 1.

Dun and Bradstreet. 2000. "Company Record View." Retrieved January 8, 2001 (http://www.dnbmdd.com/netbrs/pgate.exe).

Durkheim, Emile. [1912] 1965. *The Elementary Forms of Religious Life*. New York: The Free Press.

Dychtwald, Ken. 1999. *Age Power: How the 21st Century Will be Ruled by the New Old*. New York: Penguin Putnam Inc.

Eaton, Susan C. 2005. "Eldercare in the United States: Inadequate, Inequitable, but Not a Lost Cause." *Feminist Economics* 11(2): 37–51.

Edwards, Jennifer and J. David Knottnerus. 2007. "The Orange Order: Strategic Ritualization and Its Organizational Antecedents." *International Journal of Contemporary Sociology*. 44: 179–199.

———. 2010. "The Orange Order: Parades, Other Rituals, and Their Outcomes." *Sociological Focus* 43: 1–23.

Egger, Kim and Steve Egger. 2003. "Victims of Serial Killers: The Less-Dead." In *Victimology: A Study of Crime Victims and Their Roles*, ed. Judith Sgarzi and Jack McDevitt, 9–32. Upper Saddle River, NJ: Prentice Hall.

Elwell, Frank. 1984. "The Effects of Ownership on Institutional Services." *Gerontologist* 24: 77–83.

Etzioni, Amitai. 1961. *The Comparative Analysis of Complex Organizations*. New York: The Free Press.

———. 2000. "Toward a Theory of Public Ritual." *Sociological Theory* 18: 1.

Faber, Steve and Bob Fisher. 2005. *Wedding Crashers*. Directed by David Dobkin. New York: New Line Cinema.

Farmer, Bonnie Cashin. 1996. *A Nursing Home and Its Organizational Climate: An Ethnography*. Westport, CT: Auburn House.

Filinson, Rachel. 1995. "A Survey of Grass Roots Advocacy Organizations for Nursing Home Residents." *Journal of Elder Abuse and Neglect* 7(4): 75–84.

Foner, Nancy. 1994. *The Caregiving Dilemma: Work in an American Nursing Home*. Berkeley: University of California Press.

———. 1995. "The Hidden Injuries of Bureaucracy: Work in an American Nursing Home." *Human Organization* 54: 229–237.

Fontana, Andrea. 1977. *The Last Frontier: The Social Meaning of Growing Old.* Beverly Hills, CA: Sage Publications.

———. 1978. "Ripping off the Elderly: Inside the Nursing Home." In *Crime at the Top: Deviance in Business and Professions,* ed. John M. Johnson and Jack D. Douglas, 125–132. Philadelphia: J.B. Lipincott Company.

Forrest, Mary Brumby, Christopher B. Forrest, and Richard Forrest. 1993. *The Complete Nursing Home Guide.* Dallas: Taylor Publishing Company.

Fottler, Myron, Howard Smith, and William James. 1981. "Profits and Patient Care Quality in Nursing Homes: Are They Compatible?" *Gerontologist* 21: 532–538.

Frank, Jerome. 1936. *Law and the Modern Mind.* New York: Tudor.

Friedland, Roger and Robert R. Alford. 1991. "Bringing Society Back In: Symbols, Practices, and Institutional Contradictions." In *The New Institutionalism in Organizational Analysis,* ed. Walter W. Powell and Paul J. DiMaggio, 232–263. Chicago: The University of Chicago Press.

Fusaro, Peter C. and Ross M. Miller. 2002. *What Went Wrong at Enron?* Hoboken, NJ: John Wiley and Sons, Inc.

Gabrel, Celia. 2000. "An Overview of Nursing Home Facilities: Data from the 1997 National Nursing Home Survey. *Advanced Data for Vital and Health Statistics No. 311.* Hyattsville, MD: National Center for Health Statistics.

Gardner, Amanda. 2009. "Web Surf to Save Your Aging Brain." *HealthDay News.* Retrieved October 22, 2009 (http://www.healthday.com/Article.asp?AID=632087).

Garfinkel, Harold. 1956. "Conditions of Successful Degradation Ceremonies." *American Journal of Sociology* 61: 420–424.

Gass, Thomas Edward. 2004. *Nobody's Home: Candid Reflections of a Nursing Home Aide.* Ithaca, NY: Cornell University Press.

General Accounting Office. 2002. Report to Congressional Requesters. *Nursing Homes: More Can Be Done to Protect Residents from Abuse.* Washington, DC: GAO.

Gertz, Bill. 2002. *Breakdown: How America's Intelligence Failures Led to September 11.* Washington, DC: Regnery Publishing.

Giacalone, Joseph. 2001. *The U.S. Nursing Home Industry.* Armonk, NY: M.E. Sharpe.

Gifford-Jones, W. (aka Ken Walker). 2007. "A Feline Harbinger of Death." *The Toronto Sun,* August 11, p. 34.

Glassner, Barry. 1999. *The Culture of Fear: Why Americans Are Afraid of the Wrong Things.* New York: Basic Books.

Glenn, Evelyn Nakano. 2000. "Creating a Caring Society." *Contemporary Sociology* 29: 84–94.

Goffman, Erving. 1959. *The Presentation of Self in Everyday Life*. New York: Doubleday.

———. 1961. *Asylums*. Chicago: Aldine Publishing Company.

———. 1967. *Interaction Ritual*. New York: Pantheon Books.

Gottesman, Leonard. 1974. "Nursing Home Performance as Related to Resident Traits, Ownership Size, and Source of Payment." *The American Journal of Public Health* 64: 269–276.

Gouldner, Alvin W. 1954. *Patterns of Industrial Bureaucracy*. New York: The Free Press.

Green, Vernon L. and Deborah J. Monahan. 1981. "Structural and Operational Factors Affecting Quality of Patient Care in Nursing Homes." *Public Policy* 29: 399–415.

Greenberg, Martha. 2003. "Therapeutic Play: Developing Humor in the Nurse Patient Relationship." *The Journal of the New York State Nurses Association* 34: 25–31.

Gresham, Mary. L. 2007. "The Infantilization of the Elderly: A Developing Concept." *Nursing Forum* 15: 195–210.

Guan, Jian and J. David Knottnerus. 1999. "A Structural Ritualization Analysis of the Process of Acculturation and Marginalization of Chinese Americans." *Humboldt Journal of Social Relations* 25: 43–95.

———. 2006. "Chinatown Under Siege: Community Protest and Structural Ritualization Theory." *Humboldt Journal of Social Relations* 30: 5–52.

Gubrium, Jaber F. 1975. *Living and Dying at Murray Manor*. New York: St. Martin's Press.

———. 1993. *Speaking of Life: Horizons of Meaning for Nursing Home Residents*. New York: Aldine de Gruyter.

Hage, Jerald. 1965. "An Axiomatic Theory of Organizations." *Administrative Science Quarterly* 10: 289–320.

Hale, Sue A. 2005. *Nursing Home Diary: A Lesson in Survival*. Mustang, OK: Tate Publishing.

Hall, Richard. 1963. "The Concept of Bureaucracy: An Empirical Assessment." *American Journal of Sociology* 69: 32–40.

Hancock, Philip. 2006. "Bureaucracy." In *Encyclopedia of Social Theory*, ed. Austin Harrington, Barbara Marshall, and Hans-Peter Muller, 40–43. New York: Routledge.

Harrington, Charlene and Helen Carrillo. 1999. "The Regulation and Enforcement of Federal Nursing Home Standards, 1991–1997." *Medical Care Research and Review* December 1999: 471–494.

Hawes, Catherine and Charles D. Phillips. 1986. "The Changing Structure of the Nursing Home Industry and the Impact of Ownership on Quality Cost and Access." In *For-Profit Enterprise in Health Care,* ed. Bradford H. Gray, 492–541. Washington, DC: National Academy Press.

Help Center. 2008. "Nursing Home and Elder Abuse." *Injury Board Report.* Retrieved June 18, 2009 (http://www.injury board.com/ help-center/nursing-home-and-elder-abuse).

Henry, Jules. 1963. *Culture against Man.* New York: Random House.

Hess, John L. 1976a. "News Analysis: Nursing Homes Show Progress." *New York Times,* January 12, p. 31.

———. 1976b. "Moreland Report on Nursing Homes Cites Rockefeller." *New York Times,* February 26, p. 65.

Hochschild, Arlie R. 1983. *The Managed Heart: Commercialization of Human Feelings.* Berkeley: University of California Press.

Hodge, Paul. 1998. "National Law Enforcement Programs to Prevent, Detect, Investigate, and Prosecute Elder Abuse and Neglect in Health Care Facilities." *Journal of Elder Abuse and Neglect* 9(4): 23–42.

Hoeffer, Beverly, Karen Talerico, Joyce Rasin, Madeline Mitchell, Barbara Stewart, Darlene McKenzie, Ann Barrick, Joanne Rader, and Philip Sloane. 2006. "Assisting Cognitively Impaired Nursing Home Residents with Bathing: Effects of Two Bathing Interventions on Caregiving." *Gerontologist* 46: 524–532.

Holleman, Joey. 2009. "Zoo Employee Injured in Gorilla Escape." *The State,* June 13, p. 1.

Holmberg, R. Hopkins and Nancy N. Anderson. 1968. "Implications of Ownership for Nursing Home Care." *Medical Care* 6: 300–307.

Home, Stewart. 1989. "Toward Acognitive Culture: Steward Home Talks to Henry Flynt." *Smile,* Summer, p. 11.

Hooyman, Nancy and H. Asuman Kiyak. 1996. *Social Gerontology: A Multidisciplinary Perspective.* 4th ed. Boston, MA: Allyn and Bacon.

Horton, Paul, Gerald R. Leslie, Richard F. Larson, and Robert L. Horton. 1997. *The Sociology of Social Problems.* 12th ed. Englewood Cliffs, NJ: Prentice Hall.

Houser, Ari. 2007. "Nursing Homes: Research Report." *AARP Policy Institute Reports,* October.

Howsden, Jackie L. 1981. *Work and the Helpless Self: The Social Organization of the Nursing Home.* Lanham, MD: University Press of America.

Indo, John. 2007. "Nursing Home Neglect Adds to Health Care Nightmare." *USA Today,* December 28, p. 8A.

Jenkins, Anne and John Braithwaite. 1993. "Profits, Pressure and Corporate Lawbreaking." *Crime, Law and Social Change* 20: 221–232.

Jervis, Rick. 2007. "Trial Opens in 35 Nursing Home Deaths." *USA Today,* August 17, p. 4A.

Johnson, Carla. 2009. "Family Sues Nursing Home in Alleged Sex Attack." *The Courier,* May 13, p. 5.

Johnson, Colleen and Leslie Grant. 1985. *The Nursing Home in American Society.* Baltimore: Johns Hopkins University Press.

Johnston, Kenneth. 1993. *Busting Bureaucracy: How to Conquer Your Organization's Worst Enemy.* Homewood, IL: Business One Irwin.

Kahana, Eva. 2000. "Long-Term Care." In *The Encyclopedia of Sociology,* ed. Edgar F. Borgatta and Marie L. Borgatta, 1652–1683. New York: Macmillan.

Kahana, Eva and Sarajane Brittis. 1992. "Nursing Homes." In *The Encyclopedia of Sociology,* ed. Edgar F. Borgatta and Marie L. Borgatta, 1359–1371. New York: Macmillan.

Kane, Robert, Boris Bershadsky, Rosalie Kane, Howard Degenholtz, Jiexin Liu, Katherine Giles, and Kristen Kling. 2004. "Using Resident Reports of Quality of Life to Distinguish Among Nursing Homes." *Gerontologist* 44: 624.

Kane, Robert and Joan West. 2005. *It Shouldn't Be This Way: The Failure of Long-Term Care.* Nashville: Vanderbilt University Press.

Kayser-Jones, Jeanie. 1981. *Old, Alone, and Neglected: Care of the Aged in Scotland and the U.S.* Berkeley: University of California Press.

Kent, Zachary. 1993. *The Story of the Challenger Disaster.* Boston: Houghton Mifflin.

Kidder, Tracy. 1993. *Old Friends.* Boston: Houghton Mifflin.

Knottnerus, J. David. 1997. "The Theory of Structural Ritualization." In *Advances in Group Processes 14,* ed. Barry Markovsky, Michael J. Lovaglia, and Lisa Troyer, 257–279. Greenwich, CT: JAI Press.

———. 1999. "Status Structures and Ritualized Relations in the Slave Plantation System." In *Plantation Society and Race Relations: The Origins of Inequality,* ed. Thomas J. Durant, Jr., and J. David Knottnerus, 137–147. Westport, CT: Praeger.

———. 2002. "Agency, Structure and Deritualization: A Comparative Investigation of Extreme Disruptions of Social Order." In *Structure, Culture and History: Recent Issues in Social Theory,* ed. Sing C. Chew and J. David Knottnerus, 85–106. Lanham, MD: Rowman & Littlefield.

———. 2005. "The Need for Theory and the Value of Cooperation: Disruption and Deritualization." (Presidential Address, Mid-South

Sociological Association, Baton Rouge, 2003). *Sociological Spectrum* 25: 5–19.

———. 2009. "Structural Ritualization Theory: Application and Change." In *Bureaucratic Culture and Escalating World Problems: Advancing the Sociological Imagination,* ed. J. David Knottnerus and Bernard Phillips, 70–84. Boulder, CO: Paradigm Publishers.

———. 2010. *Ritual as a Missing Link: Sociology, Structural Ritualization Theory, and Research.* Boulder, CO: Paradigm Publishers.

Knottnerus, J. David and Phyllis E. Berry. 2002. "Spartan Society: Structural Ritualization in an Ancient Social System." *Humboldt Journal of Social Relations* 27: 1–42.

Knottnerus, J. David and David G. LoConto. 2003. "Strategic Ritualization and Ethnicity: A Typology and Analysis of Ritual Enactments in an Italian American Community." *Sociological Spectrum* 23: 425–461.

Knottnerus, J. David, David L. Monk, and Edward Jones. 1999. "The Slave Plantation System from a Total Institution Perspective." In *Plantation Society and Race Relations: The Origins of Inequality,* ed. Thomas J. Durant, Jr., and J. David Knottnerus, 17–27. Westport, CT: Praeger.

Knottnerus, J. David, and Bernard Phillips, eds. 2009. *Bureaucratic Culture and Escalating World Problems: Advancing the Sociological Imagination.* Boulder, CO: Paradigm Publishers.

Knottnerus, J. David, Jason S. Ulsperger, Summer Cummins, and Elaina Osteen. 2006. "Exposing Enron: Media Representations of Ritualized Deviance in Corporate Culture." *Crime, Media, Culture: An International Journal* 2: 177–195.

Knottnerus, J. David and Frederique Van de Poel-Knottnerus. 1999. *The Social Worlds of Male and Female Children in the Nineteenth Century French Educational System: Youth, Rituals and Elites.* Lewiston, NY: Edwin Mellen Press.

Knottnerus, J. David, Jean L. Van Delinder, and Jennifer Wolynetz. 2010. "Rituals and Power: A Cross-Cultural Case Study of Nazi Germany, the Orange Order, and Native Americans." In *Ritual as a Missing Link: Sociology, Structural Ritualization Theory, and Research,* ed. J. David Knottnerus. Boulder, CO: Paradigm Publishers.

Kobayashi, Yuka, Akiko Kaneyoshi, Atsuko Yokota, and Norito Kawakami. 2008. "Effects of a Worker Participatory Program for Improving Work Environments on Job Stressors and Mental Health among Workers: A Controlled Trial." *Journal of Occupational Health* 6: 455–470.

Koetting, Michael. 1980. *Nursing Home Organization and Efficiency: Profit Versus Non-Profit.* Lexington, MA: Lexington Books.

Lakdawalla, Darius and Tomas Philipson. 2002. "The Rise in Old-Age Longevity and the Market for Long-Term Care." *The American Economic Review* 92(1): 295–306.

Laird, Carobeth. 1979. *Limbo: A Memoir about Life in a Nursing Home by a Survivor.* Novato, CA: Chandler and Sharp.

Lee, Matthew and M. David Ermann. 1999. "Pinto 'Madness' as a Flawed Landmark Narrative: An Organization and Network Analysis." *Social Problems* 46: 30–47.

Lemke, Sonne and Rudolf H. Moos. 1986. "Quality of Residential Settings for Elderly Adults." *Journal of Gerontology* 41: 268–276.

———. 1989. "Ownership and Quality of Care in Residential Facilities for the Elderly." *Gerontologist* 29: 209–215.

Levey, Samuel, Hirsh S. Ruchlin, Bernard Stotsky, D.R. Kinloch, and W. Oppenheim. 1973. "An Appraisal of Nursing Home Care." *Journal of Gerontology* 28: 222–228.

Lewis, Ricki. 1998. "Telomere Tales." *Bioscience,* December.

Lidz, Charles, Lynn Fischer, and Robert M. Arnold.1992. *The Erosion of Autonomy in Long-Term Care.* New York: Oxford University Press.

Lopez, Steven H. 2006a. "Emotional Labor and Organized Emotional Care: Conceptualizing Nursing Home Care Work." *Work and Occupations* 33(2): 133–160.

———. 2006b. "Culture Change in Long-Term Care: A Shop-Floor View." *Politics and Society* 34: 55–80.

Lucas, Judith, Carrie Levin, Timothy Lowe, Brian Robertson, Ayse Akincigil, Usha Sambamoorthi, Scott Bilder, Eun Kwang Paek, and Stephen Crystal. 2007. "The Relationship between Organizational Factors and Resident Satisfaction with Nursing Home Care and Life." *Journal of Aging and Social Policy* 19(2): 125–151.

Lukes, Steven. 1975. "Political Ritual and Social Integration." *British Journal of Sociology* 9(2): 289–308.

Lustbader, Wendy. 2000. "The Pioneer Challenge: A Radical Change in the Culture of Nursing Homes." In *Qualities of Caring,* edited by Linda Noelker and Zev Harel. New York: Springer.

Lynch, Gerald, James Levine, Karen Terry, Margaret Smith, Michele Galietta, Maureen O'Connor, Steven Penrod, and Louis Schlesinger. 2004. "Sexual Abuse of Minors by Catholic Clergy." Special Report Prepared by the John Jay College of Criminal Justice for the United States Council of Catholic Bishops.

Mace, Nancy and Peter Rabins. 2006. *The 36-Hour Day: A Family Guide* to *Caring for People with Alzheimer Disease, Other Dementias, and Memory Loss in Later Life.* Baltimore, MD: Johns Hopkins University Press.

Managed Care Weekly. 2004. "Nursing Home Bus Kills Mental Patient." *Managed Care Weekly,* May 10.

Manning, Peter. 1977. *Police Work: The Social Organization of Policing.* Cambridge, MA: MIT Press.

Marrelli, Tina and Sandra Whittier. 2008. *Home Health Aide.* Kent Island, MD: Marrellie and Associates.

Martin, Joanne. 2002. *Organizational Culture: Mapping the Terrain.* Thousand Oaks, CA: Sage Publications.

Mayer, D. 1989. "Insider Interview: David Banks—President, Chief Operating Officer Beverly Enterprises." *Healthweek,* February 17.

McCullen, Kevin. 2000. "Elder Care Conditions Shocking." *Denver Rocky Mountain News,* August 10, p. 35A.

McKenzie, Sarah. 2000. "Sexuality in the Institutionalized Elderly." *Texas Journal on Aging* 3: 6–11.

Mehrotra, Chandra, Lisa Wagner, and Stephen Fried. 2009. *Aging and Diversity.* New York: Routledge.

Mendelson, Mary A. 1974. *Tender Loving Greed: How the Incredibly Lucrative Nursing Home Industry is Exploiting America's Old People and Defrauding Us All.* New York: Alfred Knopf.

Merton, Robert K. 1936. "The Unanticipated Consequences of Purposive Social Action." *American Sociological Review* 1: 894–904.

———. 1940. "Bureaucratic Structure and Personality." *Social Forces* 18: 560–568.

MetLife. 2006. *MetLife Market Survey of Nursing Home and Home Care Costs.* Warwick, RI: MetLife.

Metz, Ricca. 1999. *Maudie: A Positive Nursing Home Experience.* Hanover, MA: Christopher Publishing House.

Meyer, Cheryl. 2008. "Will M & A Shine on Sun Healthcare?" *The Daily Deal,* January 17.

Meyer, John W. and Brian Rowan. 1991. "Institutionalized Organizations: Formal Structure as Myth and Ceremony." In *The New Institutionalism in Organizational Analysis,* ed. Walter W. Powell and Paul J. DiMaggio, 41–62. Chicago: The University of Chicago Press.

Mills, C. Wright. 1959. *The Sociological Imagination.* NY: Oxford University Press.

Minton, Carol and J. David Knottnerus. 2008. "Ritualized Duties: The Social Construction of Gender Inequality in Malawi." *International Review of Modern Sociology* 34: 181–210.

Mitchell, Daniel. 2000. *Pensions, Politics, and the Elderly.* New York: M.E. Sharpe.

Mitra, Aditi and J. David Knottnerus. 2004. "Royal Women in Ancient India: The Ritualization of Inequality in a Patriarchal Social Order." *International Journal of Contemporary Sociology* 41: 215–231.

———. 2008. "Sacrificing Women: A Study of Ritualized Practices among Women Volunteers in India." *Voluntas: International Journal of Voluntary and Nonprofit Organizations* 19: 242–267.

Mitteness, Linda S. and Judith C. Barker. 1995. "Stigmatizing a 'Normal' Condition: Urinary Incontinence in Later Life." *Medial Anthropology Quarterly* 9: 188–210.

Mollette, Glenn. 2001. *Nursing Home Nightmares: America's Disgrace.* New York: Milo House.

Montgomery, Rhonda. 1992. "Long-Term Care." In *The Encyclopedia of Sociology,* ed. Edgar F. Borgatta and Marie L. Borgatta, 1158–1164. New York: Macmillan.

Mooney, Ruth and Maryann Greenway. 1996. *Rapid Nursing Interventions.* New York: Delmar Publishers.

Moos, Inger and Agnes Bjorn. 2006. "Use of the Life Story in Institutional Care of People with Dementia: A Review of Intervention Studies." *Ageing and Society* 26: 431–454.

Morris, Lewis. 2008. "Testimony on Nursing Homes." *In the Hands of Strangers,* House Committee on Energy and Commerce Subcommittee on Oversight and Investigations Investigation, May 15. Washington, DC.

Nachtigal, Vladimir and Marketa Votavova. 2002. "Convergence Process of Central and Eastern European Countries toward the European Union as Measured by Macroeconomic Tetragons." Prepared by the Department of Economic Policy at the University of Economics in Prague and the Macroeconomic Analysis Team of NEWTON Research Development.

Nadel, Siegfried. 1954. *Nupe Religion.* London: Routledge and Kegan Paul.

National Center for Health Statistics. 1988. *National Nursing Home Survey: 1973–1974.* Hyattsville, MD: National Center for Health Statistics.

———. 2000. *National Nursing Home Survey: 1995.* Hyattsville, MD: National Center for Health Statistics.

———. 2006. *National Nursing Home Survey: 2004.* Hyattsville, MD: National Center for Health Statistics.

Navas-Migueloa, Luis. 2008. "Testimony on Nursing Homes." *In the*

Hands of Strangers, House Committee on Energy and Commerce Subcommittee on Oversight and Investigations Investigation, May 12. Washington, DC.

NCCNHR. 2008. "History" (About the National Citizens' Coalition for Nursing Home Reform). Washington, DC: NCCNHR. Retrieved July 1, 2008 (http://nccnhr.org/public/50_541_1952.cfm).

———. 2010. "Health Care Reform Bill Will Also Improve Long-term Care." Washington, DC: NCCNHR. Retrieved June 7, 2010 (http://nccnhr.org/sites/default/files/nccnhr/documents/NCCNHR -Press-Release-on-House-Health-Reform-Vote.pdf).

Neal, Lee Ann and Julie Neal. 2000. "Nursing Home Deaths Highlight Staffing Problems." *Portland Oregonian*, April 11, p. B15.

Nerenberg, Lisa. 2002. "Abuse in Nursing Homes." *National Center on Elder Abuse Newsletter*, May.

Newman, Katherine and Cybelle Fox. 2009. "Rampage Shootings in American High School and College Settings, 2002–2008." *American Behavioral Scientist* 52: 1286–1308.

Nickerson, Colin. 2007. "With a Purr, Death Comes with Little Cat Feet." *The Boston Globe*, July 26, p. A1.

Niesz, Helga. 2005. "Nursing Home Green Houses." *OLR Research Report—2005-R-0618*. Hartford, CT: Connecticut General Assembly.

O'Brien, Mary E. 1989. *Anatomy of a Nursing Home: A New View of Residential Life*. Owings Mills, MD: National Health Publishing.

Pandya, Sheel. 2001. "Nursing Homes: Fact Sheet." *AARP Policy Institute Reports*, February.

Pareles, Jon. 2007. "The Ego Sessions: Will Success Spoil Kanye West?" *New York Times*, September 5, p. E1.

Parker, Jerrold, Herbert Waichman, and Adres Alonso. 2007. "Nursing Home Abuse and Elder Abuse Screening Problems Should be Routine in Hospitals." *PWA Articles*, September.

Paterniti, Debora. 2000. "The Micropolitics of Identity in Adverse Circumstance: A Study of Identity Making in a Total Institution." *Journal of Contemporary Ethnography* 29: 93–119.

Payne, Brian and Randy Gainey. 2006. "The Criminal Justice Response to Elder Abuse in Nursing Homes: A Routine Activities Perspective." *Western Criminology Review* 7(3): 67–81.

Pear, Robert. 2002. "Unreported Abuse Found at Nursing Homes." *New York Times*, March 3, p. 25.

———. 2008. "Serious Deficiencies in Nursing Homes Are Often Missed, Report Says." *New York Times*, May 15, p. 23.

Pelovitz, Steven. 2000. "Testimony on Nursing Home Bankruptcies."

Senate Special Committee on Aging, September 5. Washington, DC.

Perkinson, Margaret. 2003. "Defining Family Relationships in a Nursing Home Setting." In *Gray Areas: Ethnographic Encounters with Nursing Home Culture,* ed. Philip B. Stafford, 235–261. Santa Fe, NM: School of American Research Press.

Pettigrew. Andrew. 1979. "On Studying Organizational Culture." *Administrative Science Quarterly* 24: 570–581.

Phillips, Bernard. 2001. *Beyond Sociology's Tower of Babel: Reconstructing the Scientific Method.* New York: Aldine de Gruyter.

———. 2007. *Understanding Terrorism: Building on the Sociological Imagination.* Boulder, CO: Paradigm Publishers.

———. 2009. *Armageddon or Evolution? The Scientific Method and Escalating World Problems.* Boulder, CO: Paradigm Publishers.

Phillips, Bernard, and David Christner. 2009. *Saving Society: Beyond Bureaucratic Barriers to Real Solutions.* Boulder, CO: Paradigm Publishers.

Phillips, Bernard, and Louis Johnston. 2007. *The Invisible Crisis of Contemporary Society: Reconstructing Sociology's Fundamental Assumptions.* Boulder, CO: Paradigm Publishers.

Phillips, Bernard, Harold Kincaid, and Thomas J. Scheff, eds. 2002. *Toward a Sociological Imagination: Bridging Specialized Fields.* Lanham, MD: University Press of America.

Pillemer, Karl. 1988. "Maltreatment of Patients in Nursing Homes: Overview and Research Agenda." *Journal of Health and Social Behavior* 29: 227–238.

Pillemer, Karl and David Moore. 1990. "Highlights from a Study of Abuse of Patients in Nursing Homes." *Journal of Elder Abuse and Neglect* 2(1/2): 5–29.

Piller, Charles and Tim Reiterman. 2007. "After Fatal Mauling, Clues Sought on Tiger's Escape." *Los Angeles Times,* December 27, p. B1.

Powell, Lawrence, Kenneth Branco, and John Williamson. 1996. *The Senior Rights Movement: Framing the Policy Debate in America.* New York: Twayne Publishers.

Powell, Walter W. and Paul J. DiMaggio, eds. 1991. *The New Institutionalism in Organizational Analysis.* Chicago: University of Chicago Press.

Powers, Bethel. 1988a. "Social Networks, Social Support, and Elderly Institutionalized People." *Advances in Nursing Science* 10: 40–58.

———. 1988b. "Self-Perceived Health of Elderly Institutionalized People." *Journal of Cross-Cultural Gerontology* 3: 299–321.

Poxon, Joyce M. 2004. *Nursing Homes, Heaven or Hell?: A True Story of What Nursing Home Living Could Be Like for You or a Loved One.* Bloomington, IN: 1st Books Library.

Putnam, Jackson K. 1970. *Old-Age Politics in California: From Richardson to Reagan.* Stanford: Stanford University Press.

Quadagno, Jill. 2008. *Aging and the Life Course.* 4th ed. New York: McGraw-Hill.

Rabe, Gary A. and M. David Ermann. 1995. "Corporate Concealment of Tobacco Hazards: Changing Motives and Historical Contexts." *Deviant Behavior* 16: 223–44.

Ranz, Marilyn, Lanis Hicks, Victoria Grando, Gregory Petroski, Richard Madsen, David Mehr, Viki Conn, Mary Zwygart-Staffacher, Jill Scott, Marcia Flesner, Jane Bostick, Rose Porter, and Meridean Maas. 2004. "Nursing Home Quality, Cost, Staffing, and Staff Mix. *Gerontologist* 44: 24–38.

Regelson, William. 1996. *The Superhormone Promise.* New York: Simon and Schuster.

Reese, Thomas J. 2004. "Facts, Myths, and Questions." *America: The National Catholic Weekly* 190(10).

Reinhard, Susan and Robyn Stone. 2001. "Promoting Quality in Nursing Homes: The Wellspring Model." *Commonwealth Fund Research Collection.* Washington, DC: Institute for the Future of Aging Services.

Retsinas, Joan. 1986. *It's OK, Mom: The Nursing Home from a Sociological Perspective.* New York: The Tiresias Press, Inc.

Richard, Michel. 1986. "Goffman Revisited: Relatives vs. Administrators in Nursing Homes." *Qualitative Sociology* 9: 321–338.

Richardson, Hila. 1990. "Long-Term Care." In *Health Care Delivery in the United States,* ed. Anthony R. Kovner. New York: Springer.

Richardson, Virginia, Holly Dabelko, and Timothy Gregoire. 2008. "Adult Day Centers and Mental Health Care." *Social Work in Mental Health* 6(3): 41–58.

Riekse, Robert and Henry Holstege. 1996. *Growing Older in America.* New York: McGraw-Hill.

Riportella-Muller, Roberta and Doris P. Slesinger. 1982. "The Relationship of Ownership and Size to Quality of Care in Wisconsin Nursing Homes." *Gerontologist* 22: 429–434.

Ritzer, George. 2008a. *The McDonaldization of Society,* 5th ed. Los Angeles, CA: Pine Forge Press.

———. 2008b. *Sociological Theory,* 7th ed. New York: McGraw-Hill.

Rondeaux, Candace. 2007. "Bill to Identify Sex Offenders at Nursing Homes Gains Support." *The Washington Post,* January 27, p. T3.

Rosen, Anita L. and V.S. Wilbur. 1992. *Long-Term Care: Needs, Costs and Financing*. Washington, DC: Health Insurance Association of America.

Rosen, Michael. 1985. "Breakfast at Spiro's: Dramaturgy and Dominance." *Journal of Management* 11: 31–48.

Ross, Jeffrey and Stephen Richards. 2002. *Behind Bars: Surviving Prison*. Indianapolis, IN: Alpha Books.

Rothschild, Joyce and Raymond Russell. 1986. "Alternatives to Bureaucracy: Democratic Participation in the Economy." *Annual Review of Sociology* 12: 307–328.

Rowden, Tim. 1999. "Worker Charged with Assaulting Alzheimer's Patient: Nursing Home Delayed in Calling Police." *St. Louis Post Dispatch*, December 2, p. 1.

Rowles, Graham and Dallas M. High. 2003. "Family Involvement in Nursing Homes: A Decision Making Perspective." In *Gray Areas: Ethnographic Encounters with Nursing Home Culture*, ed. Philip B. Stafford, 173–202. Santa Fe, NM: School of American Research Press.

Roy, Lucinda. 2009. *No Right to Remain Silent: The Tragedy at Virginia Tech*. New York: Harmony Books.

Ryan, Michael. 2005. "Bureaucracy." In *Encyclopedia of Social Theory*, ed. George Ritzer, 71–72. Thousand Oaks, CA: Sage Publications.

Sadri, Ahmad. 1992. *Max Weber's Sociology of Intellectuals*. New York: Oxford University Press.

Sahyoun, Nadine, Laura Pratt, Harold Lentzner, Achintya Dey, and Kristen Robinson. 2001. "The Changing Profile of Nursing Home Residents" *Aging Trends No. 4*. Hyattsville, MD: National Center for Health Statistics.

Salari, Sonia. 2006. "Infantilization as Elder Mistreatment: Evidence from Five Adult Day Centers." *Journal of Elder Abuse and Neglect* 17(4): 53–91.

Sarabia, Daniel and J. David Knottnerus. 2009. "Ecological Stress and Deritualization in East Asia: Ritual Practices during Dark Age Phases." *International Journal of Sociology and Anthropology* (Open Access Online Journal) 1(1): 012–025, May. http://www.academicjournals.org/IJSA/contents/2009cont/May.htm.

Sass, James. 2000. "Emotional Labor as Cultural Performance: The Communication of Caregiving in a Nonprofit Nursing Home." *Western Journal of Communication* 64: 330–358.

Savishinsky, Joel S. 1991. *The Ends of Time: Life and Work in a Nursing Home*. New York: Bergen and Garvey.

———. 1995. "The Unbearable Lightness of Retirement: Ritual and Support in a Modern Life Passage." *Research on Aging* 17.

Scharlach, Andrew E. and Connie Frenzel. 1986. "An Evaluation of Institution-Based Respite Care." *Gerontologist* 26: 43–51.

Schnelle, John F. 2004. "Determining the Relationship Between Staffing and Quality." *Gerontologist* 44: 10–12.

Seipke, Heather. 2008. "Assisted Living, Elderly Women, and Sense of Self." *Journal of Women and Aging* 20(1/2): 131–148.

Sell, Jane, J. David Knottnerus, Christopher Ellison, and Heather Mundt. 2000. "Reproducing Social Structure in Task Groups: The Role of Structural Ritualization." *Social Forces* 79: 453–475.

Selznick, Philip. 1957. *Leadership and Administration.* Evanston, IL: Row and Peterson.

Serow, William, David Sly, and J. Michael Wrigley. 1990. *Population Aging in the United States.* New York: Greenwood Press.

Shapiro, Deanna. 2006. *Conversations at the Nursing Home: A Mother, A Daughter, and Alzheimer's.* Martinez, GA: PRA Publishing.

Shield, Renee R. 1988. *Uneasy Endings: Daily Life in an American Nursing Home.* Ithaca, NY: Cornell University Press.

Shils, Edward and Michael Young. 1953. "The Meaning of the Coronation." *Sociological Review* (n.s.) I: 63–81.

Shulman, David and Ruth Galanter. 1976. "Reorganizing the Nursing Home Industry: A Proposal." *Milbank Memorial Fund Quarterly* 54: 129–143.

Siegel, Jacob. 1993. *A Generation of Change: A Profile of America's Older Population.* New York: Russell Sage Foundation.

Silber, Gilah. 2007. *Living and Dying in a Long-Term Care Facility: Notes from a Nursing Home Doctor.* Charleston, SC: Booksurge.

Simon, David E. 1985. "Organizational Deviance: A Humanist View." *Journal of Sociology and Social Welfare* 12: 521–51.

Simons, Kelsey V. 2006. "Organizational Characteristics Influencing Nursing Home Social Service Directors' Qualifications: A National Study." *Health and Social Work* 31(4): 266–274.

Singh, Douglas and Robert Schwab. 1998. "Retention of Administrators in Nursing Homes: What Can Management Do?" *Gerontologist* 38: 362–369.

Sirrocco, Al. 1989. "Nursing Home Characteristics: 1986 Inventory of Long-Term Care Places." *Vital and Health Statistics* ser. 14, no.33, DHHS Pub. No. (PHS) 89-1828. Washington, DC: U.S. Government Printing Office.

Smith, Huston. 1992. *The Religions of Man*. New York: Harper Perennial.

Smith, Nell. 2005. "Nursing Home Litigation: Patient Died at Hands of Pathfinder, Suit by Ex-Husband Points Finger at Health Center Too." *Arkansas Democrat Gazette*, March 5, p. 1B.

Spencer, Gregory, Arnold Goldstein, and Cynthia Taeuber. 1987. *America's Centenarians: Data from the 1980 Census*, U.S. Bureau of the Census, Current Population Reports. Washington, DC: U.S. Government Printing Office.

Stafford, Philip, ed. 2003. *Gray Areas: Ethnographic Encounters with Nursing Home Culture*. Santa Fe, NM: School of American Research Press.

Stannard, Charles. 1973. "Old Folks and Dirty Work: The Social Conditions for Patient Abuse in a Nursing Home." *Social Problems* 20: 329–342.

Stone, Robyn. 1986. "Aging in the Eighties, Age 65 Years and Over—Use of Community Services." NCHS Advanced Data, no. 124. Hyattsville, MD: National Center for Health Statistics.

Stone, Robyn, Gail Cafferata, and Judith Sangl. 1987. "Caregivers of the Frail Elderly: A National Profile." *Gerontologist* 2: 616–626.

Strahan, Genevieve. 1997. "An Overview of Nursing Homes and Their Current Residents: Data from the 1995 National Nursing Home Survey." *Advanced Data for Vital and Health Statistics No. 280*. Hyattsville, MD: National Center for Health Statistics.

Terrin, Aldo. 2007. "Rite/Ritual." In *The Blackwell Encyclopedia of Sociology*, ed. George Ritzer, 3933–3936. Malden, MA: Blackwell.

Thomas, William. 1996. *Life Worth Living: How Someone You Love Can Still Enjoy Life in a Nursing Home—The Eden Alternative in Action*. Acton, MA: VanderWyk & Burnham.

Thomassen, Bjorn. 2006. "Ritual." In *Encyclopedia of Social Theory*, ed. Austin Harrington, Barbara Marshall, and Hans-Peter Muller, 522–524. New York: Routledge.

Thornburg, P. Alex, J. David Knottnerus, and Gary R. Webb. 2007. "Disaster and Deritualization: A Re-interpretation of Findings from Early Disaster Research." *The Social Science Journal* 44: 161–166.

———. 2008. "Ritual and Disruption: Insights from Early Disaster Research." *International Journal of Sociological Research* 1: 91–109.

Tisdale, Sallie. 1987. *Harvest Moon: Portrait of a Nursing Home*. New York: Henry Holt and Company.

Townsend, Claire. 1971. *Old Age: The Last Segregation*. New York: Grossman Publishers.

Treas, Judith. 1995. "Older Americans in the 1990s and Beyond." *Population Bulletin* 50: 1–47.

Trice, Harrison and Janice Beyer. 1993. *The Cultures of Work Organizations.* Englewood Cliffs, NJ: Prentice Hall.

Turner, Victor W. 1969. *The Ritual Process: Structure and Anti-Structure.* London: Routledge and Kegan Paul.

Udy, Stanley H. 1959. "Bureaucracy and Rationality in Weber's Organization Theory." *American Sociological Review* 24: 591–595.

Ulsperger, Jason S. 2002. "Geezers, Greed, Grief, and Grammar: Frame Transformation in the Nursing Home Reform Movement." *Sociological Spectrum* 22(4): 385–406.

Ulsperger, Jason S. and J. David Knottnerus. 2007. "Long-Term Care Workers and Bureaucracy: The Occupational Ritualization of Maltreatment in Nursing Homes and Recommended Policies." *Journal of Applied Social Science* 1: 52–70.

———. 2008a. "Enron: Organizational Rituals as Deviance." In *Readings in Deviant Behavior,* 5th ed., ed. Alex Thio, Thomas C. Calhoun, and Addrain Conyers, 311–314. Boston: Allyn and Bacon.

———. 2008b. "The Social Dynamics of Elder Care: Rituals of Bureaucracy and Physical Neglect in Nursing Homes." *Sociological Spectrum* 28: 357–388.

———. 2009a. "Institutionalized Elder Abuse: Bureaucratic Ritualization and Transformation of Physical Neglect in Nursing Homes." In *Bureaucratic Culture and Escalating World Problems: Advancing the Sociological Imagination,* ed. J. David Knottnerus and Bernard Phillips, 134–155. Boulder, CO: Paradigm Publishers.

———. 2009b. "Illusions of Affection: Bureaucracy and Emotional Neglect in Nursing Homes." *Humanity and Society* 33: 238–257.

Ulsperger, Jason S. and John Paul. 2002. "The Presentation of Paradise: Impression Management and the Contemporary Nursing Home." The Qualitative Report 7(4). Retrieved June 5, 2009 (http://www.nova.edu/ssss/QR/QR7-4/ulsperger.html).

Ulsperger, Jason S. and Kristen Kloss Ulsperger. 2001. "Profit, Ownership, and the Corporation: Deviance in American Elder Care." *Free Inquiry in Creative Sociology* 29: 5–9.

———. 2002. "Structural Consensus, Deviance, and Elder Care: A Content Analysis of Newspaper Articles." *Southwestern Mass Communication Journal* 18(1): 12–21.

Ulsperger, Jason S, Kristen Kloss Ulsperger, and Cole Smith. 2009. *River Valley Reflections: Heritage from the Halls of Long-Term Care.* Bloomington, IN: Xlibris.

U.S. Bureau of Census. 1993. "Current Population Reports, Special Studies." *Sixty-five Plus in America*. Washington, DC: U.S. Government Printing Office.

U.S. Federation of Worker Cooperatives. 2009. *About Worker Cooperatives*. Retrieved October 22, 2009 (http://www.usworker.coop/aboutworkercoops).

Van de Poel-Knottnerus, Frederique and J. David Knottnerus. 1994. "Social Life Through Literature: A Suggested Strategy for Conducting a Literary Ethnography." *Sociological Focus* 27: 67–80.

————. 2002. *Literary Narratives on the Nineteenth and Early Twentieth-Century French Elite Educational System: Rituals and Total Institutions*. Lewiston, NY: Edwin Mellen Press.

Van Gennep, Arnold. ([1908] 1960). *The Rites of Passage*. London: Routledge and Kegan Paul.

Varner, Monica K. and J. David Knottnerus. 2002. "Civility, Rituals and Exclusion: The Emergence of American Golf During the Late Nineteenth and Early Twentieth Centuries." *Sociological Inquiry* 72: 426–441.

Vaughan, Diane. 1992. "Regulating Risk: Implications of the Challenger Accident." In *Organizations, Uncertainties, and Risk*, ed. James F. Short, Jr. and Lee Clarke, 235–253. Boulder, CO: Westview Press.

————. 1999. "The Dark Side of Organizations: Mistakes, Misconduct, and Disaster." *Annual Review of Sociology* 25: 271–305.

Vesperi, Maria. 1983. "The Reluctant Consumer: Nursing Home Residents in the Post-Bergman Era." In *Growing Old in Different Societies: Cross-Cultural Perspectives*, ed. Jay Sokolovsky, 225–237. Belmont, CA: Wadsworth Publishing Company.

————. 2003. "The Use of Irony in Contemporary Ethnographic Narrative." In *Gray Areas: Ethnographic Encounters with Nursing Home Culture*, ed. Philip B. Stafford, 69–102. Santa Fe, NM: School of American Research Press.

Vladeck, Bruce C. 1980. *Unloving Care: The Nursing Home Tragedy*. New York: Basic Books.

Vold, George B., Thomas J. Bernard, and Jeffery B. Snipes. 2002. *Theoretical Criminology*, 5th ed. New York: Oxford University Press.

Wallbank, Walter, Alastair M. Taylor, Nels M. Bailkey, George F. Jewsbury, Clyde J. Lewis, and Neil J. Hackett. 1992. *Civilization Past & Present*, 7th ed. New York: HarperCollins.

Warner, Gene. 1999. "Aide Charged in Death at Nursing Home." *Buffalo News*, November 24, p. B1.

Warner, W. Lloyd. 1959. *The Living and the Dead: A Study of the Symbolic*

Life of Americans (Yankee City Series). New Haven, CT: Yale University Press.

———. 1962. *American Life: Dream and Reality.* Revised Edition. Chicago: University of Chicago Press.

Weber, Max. 1946. *From Max Weber: Essays in Sociology.* Trans., ed., and introduced by Hans Gerth and C. Wright Mills. New York: Oxford University Press.

Weems, Kerry. 2008. "Testimony on Nursing Homes." *In the Hands of Strangers,* House Committee on Energy and Commerce Subcommittee on Oversight and Investigations Investigation, May 15. Washington, DC.

Weiner, Audrey S. and Judah L. Ronch. 2003. *Culture Change in Long-Term Care.* New York: Haworth Social Work Practice Press.

Weisbrod, Burton A. and Mark Schlesinger. 1983. *Public, Private, Nonprofit Ownership and the Response to Asymmetric Information: The Case of Nursing Homes.* Discussion paper No. 209, Center for Health Economics and Law, University of Wisconsin at Madison.

Whitmer, Rachel and Susan Whitbourne. 1997. "Evaluation of Infantilizing Speech in a Rehabilitation Setting." *International Journal of Aging and Human Development* 44(2): 129–136.

Wiener, Joshua and David Stevenson.1998. "Repeal of the Boren Amendment: Implications for Quality of Care in Nursing Homes." New Federalism: Issues and Options for States series, No. A-30. Washington, DC. Urban Institute. Retrieved July 1, 2008 (http://www.urban.org/publications/308020.html).

Williams, Ann. 1999. "An Association is Born." *Provider* January: 40–42.

Williams, Linda. 1984. "The Classic Rape: When Do Victims Report?" *Social Problems* 31(4): 459–467.

Williams, Rachael. 2005. "Nursing Homes in Filthy State." *Birmingham Post,* September 13, p. 6.

Williamson, Molly. 2006. "Nursing Home Trial Nears End." *The State Journal,* May 4, p. 1.

Winn, Sharon. 1974. "Analysis of Selected Characteristics of a Matched Sample of Non-profit and Proprietary Nursing Homes in the State of Washington." *Medical Care* 12: 221–228.

Wu, Yanhong and J. David Knottnerus. 2005. "Ritualized Daily Practices: A Study of Chinese 'Educated Youth.'" *Shehui (Society)* (6): 167–185.

———. 2007. "The Origins of Ritualized Daily Practices: From Lei Feng's Diary to Educated Youth's Diaries." *Shehui (Society)* (1): 98–119.

Yetter, Deborah. 2006. "Law Sought on Nursing Home Staff Levels." *The Courier-Journal,* June 5, p. 1.

Zarit, Steve H., Pamela A. Todd, and Judy M. Zarit. 1986. "Subjective Burden of Husbands and Wives as Caregivers: A Longitudinal Study." *Gerontologist* 26: 260–266.

Zhang, Xinzhi and David C. Grabowski. 2004. "Nursing Home Staffing and Quality Under the Nursing Home Reform Act." *Gerontologist* 44: 13–23.

INDEX

✳

ABOUT THE AUTHORS

Jason S. Ulsperger is Assistant Professor of Sociology at Arkansas Tech University. He received his master's degree from Arkansas State University and Ph.D. from Oklahoma State University, where he won the O. D. Duncan Award for his academic and professional service. For years, he has been a volunteer in nursing homes throughout the southern United States. He teaches courses in sociology, criminal justice, and gerontology. He is the author of multiple articles on nursing home law, elder abuse, and nursing home reform. He is also heading an ongoing project involving the collection of oral histories from elders in the Arkansas River Valley. He and J. David Knottnerus recently won the Mid-South Sociological Association's Sociological Spectrum Award for their article, "The Social Dynamics of Elder Care." His other recent articles appear in *Crime, Media, Culture: An International Journal, Applied Social Science,* and *Humanity and Society.*

J. David Knottnerus is Professor of Sociology at Oklahoma State University. He received his Ph.D. from Southern Illinois

University–Carbondale. He teaches classes in social psychology, theory, and inequality/social structure. He is currently working on a number of projects utilizing structural ritualization theory. Recent books include *Ritual as a Missing Link: Sociology, Structural Ritualization Theory and Research; American Golf and the Development of Civility: Rituals of Etiquette in the World of Golf* (with Monica K. Varner); *Bureaucratic Culture and Escalating World Problems: Advancing the Sociological Imagination* (co-edited with Bernard Phillips); *Structure, Culture and History: Recent Issues in Social Theory* (co-edited with Sing C. Chew); and *Literary Narratives on the Nineteenth and Early Twentieth-Century French Elite Educational System: Rituals and Total Institutions* (with Frederique Van de Poel–Knottnerus).